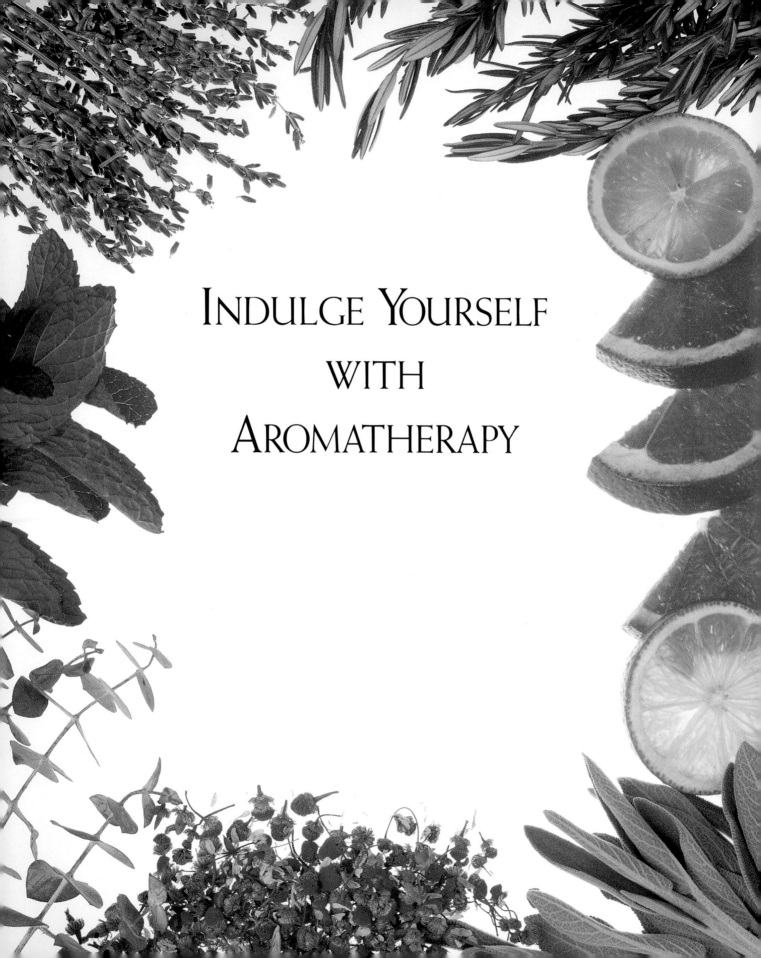

Indulge Yourself with Aromatherapy

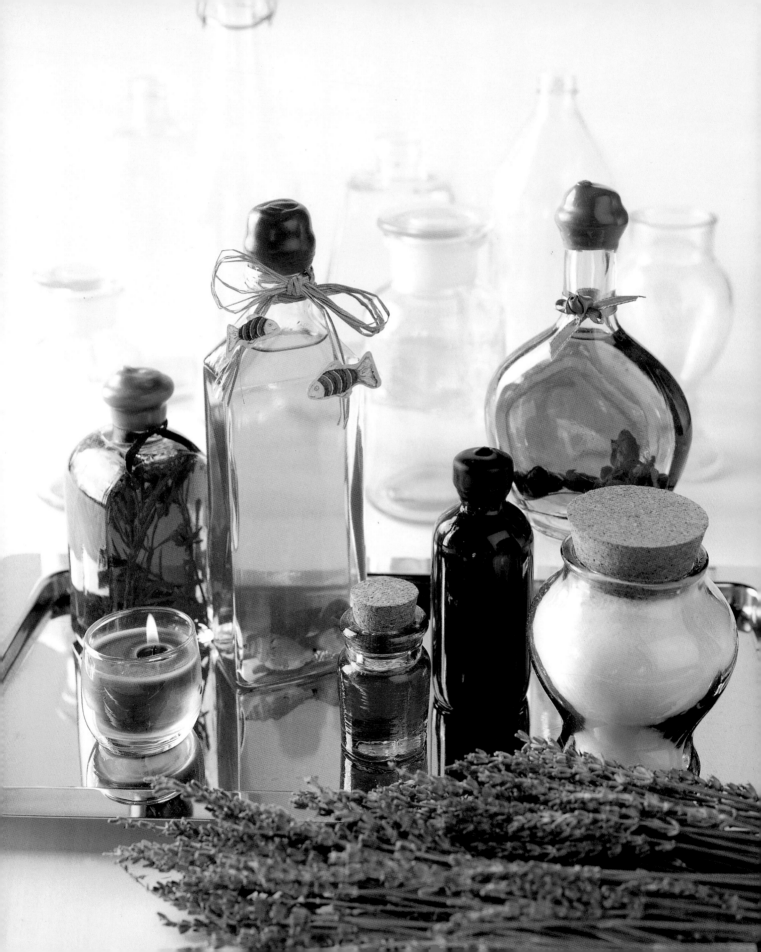

INDULGE YOURSELF
WITH
AROMATHERAPY

M. Lou Luchsinger

Sterling Publishing Co., Inc.
New York

Prolific Impressions
Production Staff:

Editor: Mickey Baskett
Graphics: Dianne Miller, Karen Turpin
Styling: Laney Crisp McClure
Photography: Pat Molnar, Jerry Mucklow
Illustrations: Jill Lampe
Administration: Jim Baskett

CAUTION: Remedies are intended to enhance your lifestyle, and not intended to take the place of advice or treatment from your physician. If you are seriously ill, please consult your physician. Do not take remedies internally. Young children, pregnant women, or persons under a doctor's care should consult their physician before using essential oils.

Library of Congress Cataloging-in-Publication Data Available

Luchsinger, M. Lou.
   Indulge yourself with aromatherapy / M. Lou Luchsinger.
     p. cm.
   Includes index.
   ISBN 0-8069-2763-1
    1. Aromatherapy--Popularworks. 1. Title.

RM666.A68 L83 2000
615'.321--dc21
                                    00-033901

Published by Sterling Publishing Company, Inc.
387 Park Avenue South, New York, N.Y. 10016
Produced by Prolific Impressions, Inc.
160 South Candler St., Decatur, GA 30030
©2000 Prolific Impressions, Inc.
Distributed in Canada by Sterling Publishing
c/o Canadian Manda Group, One Atlantic Avenue, Suite 105
Toronto, Ontario, Canada M6K 3E7
Distributed in Great Britain and Europe by Cassell PLC
Wellington House, 125 Strand, London WC2R 0BB, England
Distributed in Australia by Capricorn Link (Australia) Pty. Ltd.
P.O. Box 6651, Baulkham Hills, Business Centre, NSW 2153 Australia

Printed in Hong Kong

Sterling ISBN 0-8069-2763-1

About the Author
M. Lou Luchsinger

Lou Luchsinger is a former high school English teacher, college professor and administrator. In her present career, she owns a farm in the rolling countryside of Pennsylvania with her husband Vince, growing Christmas trees and timber trees. This idyllic, natural setting fostered Lou's fascination with herbs and dried flowers. For the past eight years, she has spent time researching and experimenting, and finally specializing in aromatherapy, herbs, and dried flowers (many of which she grows on her farm).

Lou has had her own retail shop where she sold her specially made herbal cosmetics and dried flower creations. Always the educator, she enjoys speaking to garden clubs and other civic groups about all the wonderful uses of herbs and aromatherapy. She also practices what she preaches, and enjoys the year-round benefits of the aromatherapy gifts that her herbs and plants release to her.

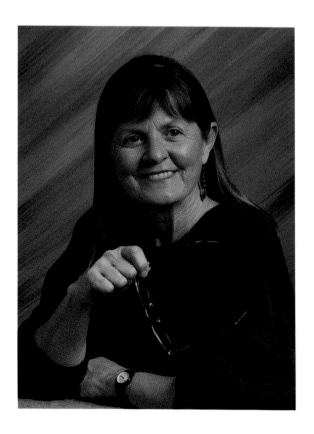

CONTENTS

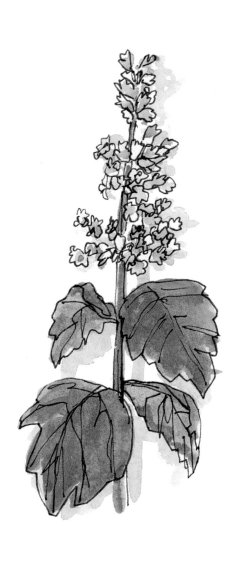

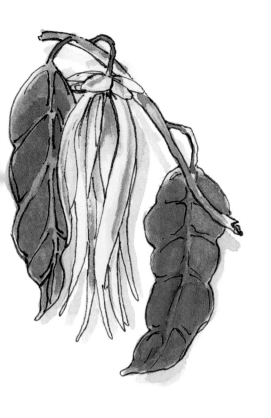

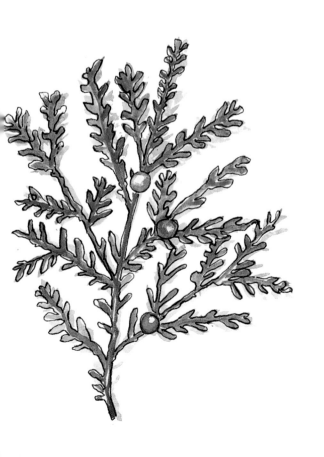

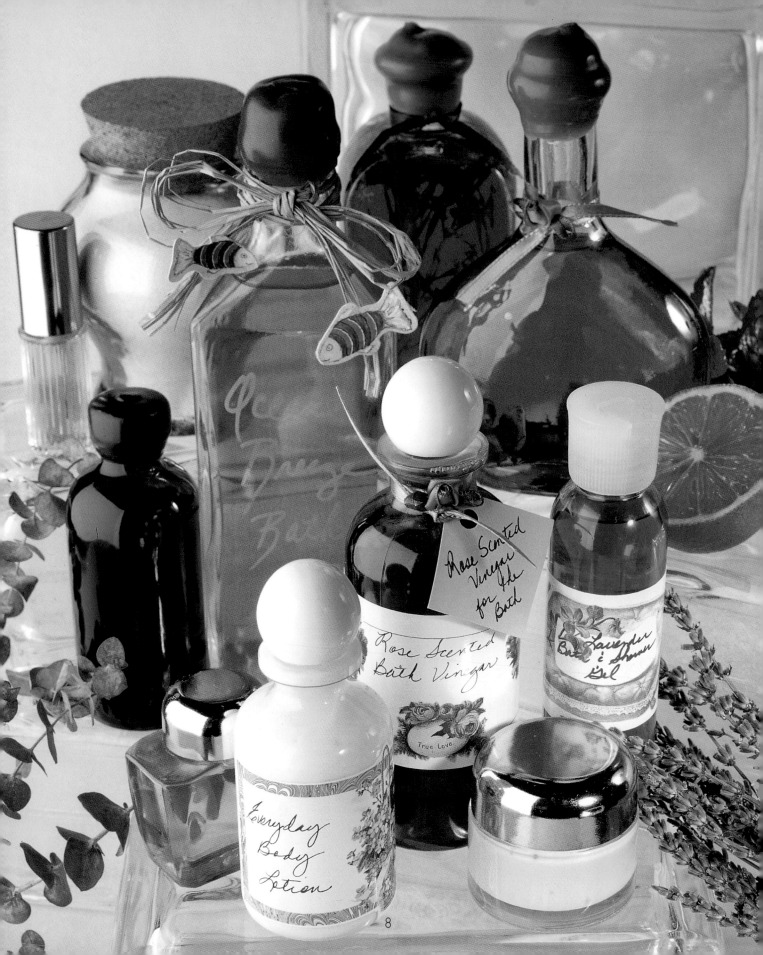

Rose Scented
Vinegar for the Bath

Rose Scented
Bath Vinegar

True Love.

Lavender
Bath & Shower
Gel

Everyday
Body
Lotion

8

INTRODUCTION

As I write this, I have the scent of eucalyptus wafting around me. It's helping me to breathe better, invigorating my creative juices, and giving my thoughts clarity while cleansing the air of negative energy. That's a pretty tall order for any scent to fill, but essential oils aren't just scents. They are the spirit of the plant, nature's gift to mankind, and through them many wonderful experiences are realized.

I first began working with essential oils about 7 years ago. Some friends of mine were having a crafts fair in their home and wanted a speaker to talk about some aspect of herbs. I had already spoken for them on other occasions on cooking with herbs and crafting with herbs so I had to search for a new idea. While browsing through some of my herbal magazines, I found "herbal cosmetics," lotions, creams and other wonderful concoctions for the body made by using natural products and essential oils. I thought this was a wonderful idea for a presentation. By

If this is your first book on aromatherapy and your first time using essential oils, your olfactory system may feel overloaded. Essential oils are powerful, potent, and can overwhelm the novice nose. But stick with your experiment. Once you have really smelled what lavender, rose, lemon smells like, you will be unable to settle for less than the purity of essential oils. You will learn what the oils can do for you and you will look for ways to include them in everything you do. You may - as I have - look for recruits. I now have friends and family asking for bottles of essential oils and the special concoctions that they have found works in ways products without essential oils cannot. My mom who suffered her second stroke in June, 1999, now uses lavender oil everyday on her temples, preventing the debilitating headaches associated with her stroke from returning. She uses it at night to help calm her for sleeping. My husband keeps a bottle of basil oil in his car for late night trips back from the

"Aromatherapy is not merely an indulgence,
but a way of life, one that you deserve."

reading a number of books and experimenting, I began on a road that led not only to the presentation, where I had more than 50 different herbal cosmetic products to show - and sell - but also to beginning a business that included dried flower arrangements and herbal cosmetics, first by special order then by having my own retail shop.

At the beginning of my journey, I knew nothing about essential oils. Along the way, I have experienced the power of essential oils and am a true believer in their wonderful - and necessary - addition to our lives. I continue to learn which oils work best for me; I use my own cosmetics or buy those that have essential oils in them. I have lavender oil in bottles located throughout the house, ready for easy access to treat burns, headaches and to lift spirits. No longer will I settle for scent alone - as in fragrance oils; I want and need the accompanying health benefits of essential oils.

university where he works. He says sniffing the oil keeps him alert.

If this book is one of your collection of books on aromatherapy and essential oils, I hope you find it full of interesting ideas that will add to your knowledge base. I have collected many books on the subject and usually find something of value in each of them.

I wish for you a pleasant, rewarding journey as you enter the world of aromatherapy. You may find it changes your life forever - you will soon learn that aromatherapy is not merely an indulgence, but a way of life, one that you deserve. Experiment and find YOUR oils, the ones that make a difference in your health and well-being. They're just waiting to become part of your daily life.

WHAT IS AROMATHERAPY?

Aromatherapy is a modern term for a healing art that is ages old. Its earliest use was in China as early as 4000 B.C. The Chinese were probably the first to use essential oils for medicinal purposes. The Egyptians were known for using aromatics in rituals and healing, including different forms of massage, and for cosmetics and embalming. Many of their formulas were carved into the stone walls of Egyptian temples so that we have been able to document their widespread use of essential oils. However, the first herbal/medicinal handbook describing numerous uses for plant oils was not published until the 17th century. Chemical substitutes became popular in the 19th century and almost halted the use of pure and natural oils.

It was not until 1928 that the term "aromatherapy" was coined by Rene-Maurice Gattefossé, a French chemist working in his family's perfumier business. At first his research was confined to the cosmetic uses of essential oils,

offer aromatherapy massage and products to their clients.

Aromatherapy is a way to improve the quality of life on a physical, emotional and spiritual level. The basis of aromatherapy is the use of essential oils, the vital life essence of aromatic plants and flowers in a concentrated form.

Not all plants contain essential oils; less than 20% have essences. In those that do - more than 150 – the oil, or essence, is contained in highly specialized glands that are present in the foliage, flower, or other plant material. In fact, roots, stalks, bark, leaves, flowers, blossoms, seeds, nuts, fruits and resins have all been used to obtain the plant oil. In the plant, the essential oil is part of the plants own immune system. As the oils evaporate, they create a barrier around the leaf or other plant part, and so reduce water loss through evaporation in the plant itself. Essential oils in essence appear to provide some defense against infection in the plant

"Aromatherapy is a way to improve the quality of life on a physical, emotional and spiritual level."

but he soon realized that many oils also had powerful antiseptic properties. He became fascinated with the therapeutic possibilities of the oils after discovering by accident that lavender was able to heal a severe burn on his hand quite rapidly and help prevent scarring. He went on to treat many burn victims in WWII and continued his research on the healing properties of essential oils.

Following Gattefossé's research into the properties of essential oils, a great deal of interest was generated in France and Italy. Not only were oils found to heal skin and strengthen immunity, but they were also capable of relieving mental conditions such as anxiety and depression.

Over the last 25 years an increasing number of books have been written on aromatherapy and even though Americans have not fully embraced the power of essential oils in their everyday lives as most Europeans have, more attention is being paid to aromatherapy's contribution to health and well-being. Some hotels, airports, and resort areas now

material, helping to strengthen its immune system, and attract insects that are vital to pollination. The plants that contain essential oils are found mainly in hot, dry habitats. At certain times of the day, and particular times of the year, the essential oils are present at optimum levels, and this is the best time for harvest and distillation. The amount of oil produced by a plant is also affected by the growing conditions, including the type of soil, the amount of sunlight it receives, and rainfall. Many plants are needed to produce even an ounce of oil - for example, 6 pounds of lavender flowers are needed to make 1 oz of oil while 300 pounds of rose petals are required for 1 oz. of rose oil.

Most essential oils are obtained through steam distillation. This process involves filling large vats with plant material which is then steamed at high pressure. The hot steam causes the essential oils to be released by the plant. The oils do not dissolve in water and will float to the top. They are then skimmed from the top. These pure "life forces" of the plant are then available to use in many different ways. They are highly concentrated and have a unique chemical composition consisting of botanical vitamins, hormones and antibiotics. In comparison to dried herbs, essential oils are 75-100 times more concentrated. Since they are the most potent part of the plant, only a small amount is needed to be effective.

Essential oils have a consistency similar to that of water, and most are lighter than water. All of them differ from vegetable oils in that they are not greasy. Most are colorless. They are extremely volatile, which means they will quickly evaporate when exposed to air.

The action of an essential oil on the body is holistic, combining both physical and mental aspects. Essential oils work together with all aspects of the body, strengthening rather than weakening it so that it may aid in the healing and restorative process.

Essential oils are extremely flexible in their applications. Their ability to affect people on so many different levels - physical, emotional, psychological - is a special element unmatched by other healing arts. You can easily incorporate them into many of your daily activities. Pure essential oils have a place in every home and every lifestyle. They are nature's alternative to the many synthetic chemicals that have invaded our lives and homes in the names of health, cleanliness, and environmental enhancement.

HOW CAN AROMATHERAPY IMPROVE HEALTH AND WELL-BEING?

Nature creates essential oils from basic hydrocarbon molecules. The type of molecules that make up the essential oil determines the range of effects the oil will have. Some oils have up to 250 different components making them nearly impossible to duplicate synthetically. These aromatic molecules of essential oils come in contact with the only part of our brain that is exposed outside our body - the olfactory bulb. This olfactory bulb, which is responsible for the sense of smell, is 10,000 times more sensitive than any other sense. Scents are tied directly to the neo-cortex of the brain which is the part that processes memory and emotions and where basic drives are stimulated. By breathing essential oils, you elicit all kinds of responses which promote a sense of health and well-being. It is believed the molecules of an essential oil also permeate the skin and are carried by the lymphatic and circulatory systems to the inner organs. Whether the oil is absorbed through the skin or inhaled, once in the bloodstream and body fluids, it works therapeutically, however small the dose.

The chemicals in essential oils unlock the body's ability to heal. Essential oils are able to influence all aspects of the body's functions, from tissues to organs, to body fluids and cells, as well as the emotional state and the spiritual aspects of the person.

The results of aromatherapy are very individual; no two persons are affected by the same essential oil in exactly the same way. Even the same person can be affected differently by the same oil depending on surroundings, time of day, or mood.

The idea behind aromatherapy is, first, to find the scents, unique for each individual, that evoke positive sensory feelings and emotions, and then to introduce those scents into our everyday life to enhance well-being. Natural scents keep us connected to the earth – grounded – sparking memories and emotions and healing the spirit.

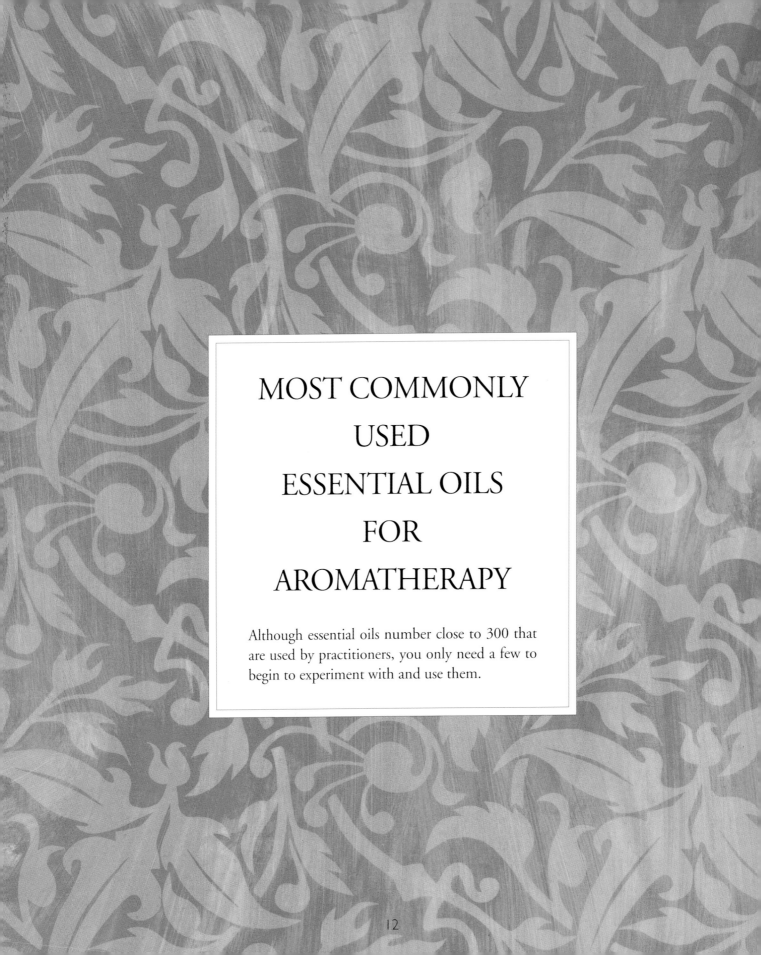

MOST COMMONLY
USED
ESSENTIAL OILS
FOR
AROMATHERAPY

Although essential oils number close to 300 that are used by practitioners, you only need a few to begin to experiment with and use them.

Following is a description of 16 oils that may be useful for a diversity of purposes, followed by 3 of the most expensive essential oils. You may decide to start with only one. If you're planning to use the recipes in this book, you may need 3-4 to begin. Find the ones that fit your needs, that smell the best to you, that will serve a particular purpose. Take your time to learn about each one and its effect on you. Remember, essential oils are very personal; they affect each of us in different ways. The descriptions serve as a way to begin your search for the oils that you would like to include in your everyday life. I have listed them in order of my favorites, beginning with the one I use most.

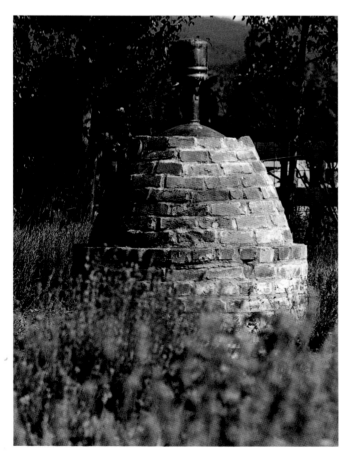

Shown here is a replica of a 14th century-style still. This type of still was used by Benedictine monks of England to extract oil from lavender. They are reported to be the first people to commercialize essential oils. This replica can be seen at Leighvander Cottage, in Blenheim, New Zealand. This delightful lavender garden is owned and operated by Elsie & Brian Hall. Elsie uses the still for demonstrations during tours of her intoxicating garden, although most of the oil from her lavender plants is extracted commercially. At Leighvander Cottage you can purchase lavender plants, pure essential lavender oil, and products made from the oil such as hand creams, lip gloss, and bath oils.

Lavender

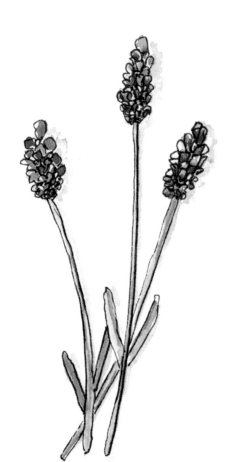

If you could buy only one oil, this would be the one! Lavender essential oil is a multi-purpose oil and is one of the most used essential oils in aromatherapy because of its diverse nature. The essential oil is distilled from the leaves, flowers, and stems of the plant.

Lavender has a long history. The Pharaohs of Egypt used the pure oil as a fragrance, and the Romans bathed in lavender water. In England it was commonly used to scent linen boxes, as an aid to controlling insects. It has always been used in perfume and cosmetics since it blends so well with other essential oils.

Lavender is the oil most associated with healing skin irritations because it stimulates the cells of injured skin to heal quickly and smoothly. It is wonderful to use on sunburn and is excellent for skin care in general because it suits all skin types. It can be useful for eczema, psoriasis, burns, cuts and wounds, abscesses and ulcers.

Lavender has many traditional therapeutic uses. It can be helpful for colds and bronchitis, for rheumatic pain, muscle spasms, balancing blood pressure, and not least, as a sedative to the central nervous system, for headaches, relieving tension and anxiety, mild depression and insomnia. It's a lovely oil for baths, for air fresheners, or simply for putting on a tissue and breathing in its lovely aroma. A major plus for this oil is that it can be used "neat," or undiluted directly on the skin. It is one of the few oils that can be used in this manner.

Properties: Balancing, soothing, clarifying, normalizing, cleansing
Blends well with: eucalyptus, geranium, jasmine, ylang ylang, lemon, orange, rose

Tea Tree

This essential oil is distilled from the leaves of the Australian and New Zealand tea tree. In New Zealand it is called "Manuka." The common English name is "tea tree" because it was brewed as a tea substitute by early English settlers of New Zealand. Tea tree oil is another gentle oil that can be used neat, placing directly on cuts to clean, disinfect, and alleviate pain. It is invaluable in a first aid kit for use as an antiseptic in treatment of cuts, fungus, and infection. Tea tree oil is extremely effective in aiding the immune system, helping the body to fight disease. It has a spicy, medicinal aroma. Tea tree is one of the most scientifically researched oils.

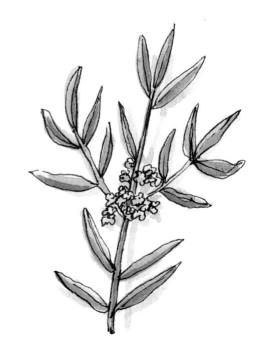

Properties: Anti-inflammatory, antiseptic, antiviral
Blends well with: eucalyptus, clary sage, lavender, lemon, rosemary, ylang ylang

Eucalyptus

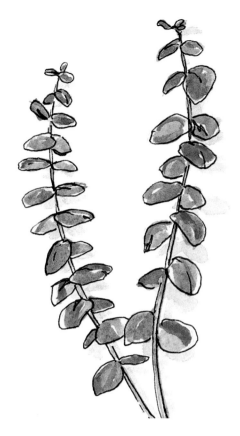

Eucalyptus is one of the most well-known oils, easily recognizable by its camphoric scent. This Australian native, distilled from the leaves of a tall tree, is an extremely versatile oil that helps refresh the body, builds the immune system, and protects it during the winter. This oil has a deeply grounding quality which can help cool overheated emotions. Its cleansing and harmonizing nature makes it useful for places where there has been emotional or physical conflict and for places that just feel uncomfortable. Its powerful head clearing ability makes eucalyptus highly effective in relieving congestion. This same head clearing ability can also aid concentration. The oil deeply penetrates and relieves tired, stiff, sore muscles and joints. It can be used as an antidote to bites and stings. Eucalyptus has a place in every household. Its antiseptic qualities are invaluable in purifying and clearing the air, making it an excellent oil for sick rooms.

Properties: Purifying, invigorating, balancing, cooling
Blends well with: bergamot, juniper, lavender, lemon, rosemary

Roman Chamomile

Chamomile was a sacred herb of the Saxons. This essential oil has been in use for over 2000 years as a natural treatment for nervous conditions and insomnia. This gentle oil has long been used for its calming effect, especially on hyperactive children. In skin care, chamomile is useful for soothing irritated skin and is very effective in steam facials or cold compresses. The oil has a sweet, fruit aroma, likened to an apple smell. The essence comes from the freshly dried white flowers of the herb. The essential oil is very effective as a headache remedy, a soothing bath addition, a tranquil, diffused scent for the home.

Properties: Sedative, anti-inflammatory, antiseptic
Blends well with: bergamot, clary sage, geranium, jasmine, lavender, patchouli, rose, ylang ylang

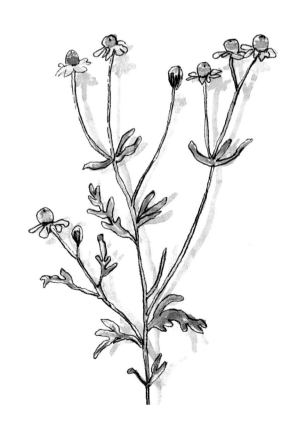

Juniper

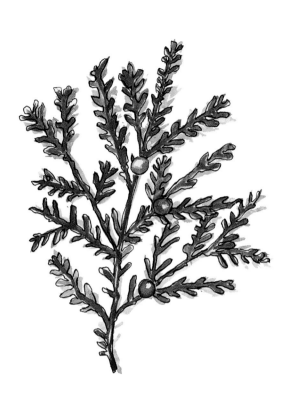

For improved overall health, juniper is a must for the home shelf. It is believed to be antiseptic, astringent, diuretic, cleansing, detoxifying, antispasmodic, parasiticidal, and anti-rheumatic. Juniper is useful in skin care preparations as well. Juniper, as an antiseptic, has long been employed to clean and disinfect. When added to cleaning water, it purifies a home and leaves a clean, woodsy scent. Juniper is the plant of protection, having been used throughout the ages as a spiritual and bodily protector. In Britain, juniper was once hung on the front doors of houses to keep away witches on the eve of May, and its wood was frequently burned to banish demons. The essential oil is obtained from the ripe, blue juniper berries, which are also an important ingredient in giving it its distinctive flavor. Its aroma blends well with other oils. The essential oil can help to clear a burdened mind, building up emotional reserves. An excellent diuretic, juniper can help to cleanse the body of toxins, and speed recovery in convalescence. It can act as a sedative when used in small doses, and as a stimulant when the dosage is increased.

CAUTION: Juniper oil should not be used in the first trimester of pregnancy or by those who have kidney problems since it may prove too stimulating.

Properties: Cleansing, detoxifying, antiseptic, strengthening
Blends well with: bergamot, clary sage, geranium, rosemary, sandalwood

Peppermint

Peppermint is a perennial herb that is cultivated throughout the world. Its medicinal qualities were widely appreciated by the Ancient Egyptians, Chinese, and Indians. The Romans used to crown themselves with peppermint wreaths during feasts in order to take advantage of its detoxifying effects. Peppermint is a favorite of many people. It is piercing and pungent. This oil is both cooling and refreshing on the skin and extremely versatile for home use. Its head clearing aroma is stimulating and helps to overcome fatigue. Peppermint aids concentration and decisiveness. Peppermint has been found to be uplifting and rejuvenating. The essential oil has been found effective in cases of headaches, congestion, fever, fatigue, and muscle soreness.

CAUTION: Because the oil is so strong, it must ALWAYS be properly diluted before using.

Properties: Uplifting, rejuvenating, antiseptic, stimulating, clearing
Blends well with: lemon, eucalyptus, rosemary, rosewood, juniper

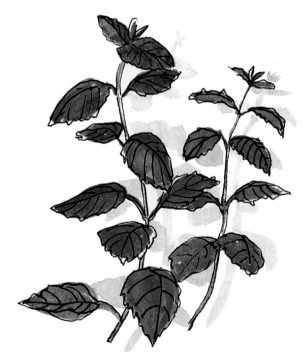

Rosemary

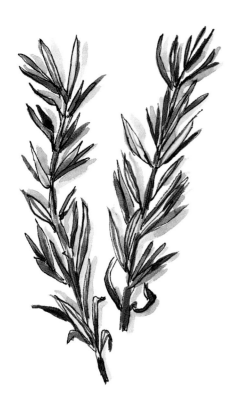

Rosemary is the "I remember" oil. The herb is a shrubby evergreen bush cultivated in most parts of the world but native to the Mediterranean region. It has scented, silver-grey, needle-like leaves and pale lilac or blue flowers, from which the oil is distilled. In Ancient Greece it was burned in shrines, and in Ancient Rome it was regarded as a symbol of regeneration. The Moors planted it around their orchards as an insect repellent, and it was used in the Middle Ages as a fumigant to drive away evil spirits. More recently, the French used it as a disinfectant in hospital wards during epidemics. This necessary essential oil enhances mental clarity, concentration, memory, and creativity. Rosemary essential oil can provide a much needed lift during a long day with its stimulating aroma. Rosemary has been found to ease stiff, aching, tired, or overworked muscles when used after activity as a massage or bath oil. It is a wonderful oil for the hair, keeping it shiny and healthy. Rosemary rejuvenates the skin. This oil is a good addition for all first aid kits since it has antiseptic properties and is excellent for wounds and burns. CAUTION: Can be irritating to skin so must be properly diluted. Also, people with epilepsy or asthma should be cautious in their use of this oil since it has a very strong scent.

Properties: Clarifying, warming, invigorating, antiseptic
Blends well with: frankincense, geranium, lemon, juniper, eucalyptus

Geranium

This adaptable oil has been widely used since antiquity when it was thought to keep evil spirits at bay. The plant is native to Africa but is now cultivated in many parts of the world as a house plant as well as commercially for its oil. The scented geranium plant has a very fragrant leaf from which this essential oil is obtained. The oil is a balancer for the body, mind, and emotions. It eases anxiety, apprehension, depression, mood swings, and emotional imbalance. Geranium oil is a must for many women who need help balancing during those up and down hormonal times. It encourages harmonious relationships and has a normalizing effect, either stimulating or sedating according to individual needs. Geranium essence is used frequently in perfumes and soaps, being a good addition to skin care since it suits all skin types. It is particularly effective for sluggish, oily complexions and combination skin.

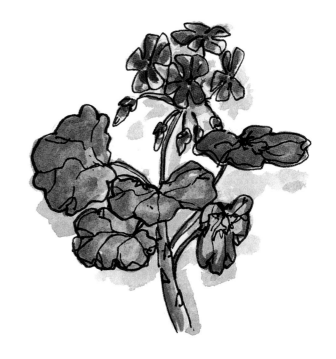

Properties: Anti-fungal, antiseptic, antidepressant, uplifting, balancing
Blends well with: bergamot, clary sage, jasmine, juniper, lavender, patchouli, roman chamomile, rose, rosemary, sandalwood

Bergamot

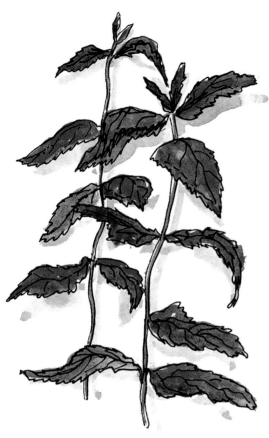

This wonderfully refreshing and renewing oil is expressed from the peel of the bergamot fruit grown in Southern Italy and some parts of Africa. Bergamot leaves are used in Earl Grey tea. The essential oil acts primarily on the nervous system where it can both soothe and invigorate. It is a bright, cheerful, uplifting oil, used when an individual feels depressed or anxious. At times of stress, just smelling the oil will do wonders for your confidence. The uplifting nature of this oil helps the grief-stricken to be more open to the positive, healing effects of joy and love. It promotes confidence, courage, and discernment. Women benefit greatly from this essential oil since it helps regulate the menstrual cycle and relieves PMS as well as easing symptoms of menopause. Bergamot cools fevers and has been used in the treatment of urinary tract infections. It can also soothe the digestive and respiratory system, encouraging appetite and a return to health during convalescence. The oil is also effective against travel sickness. With its regenerative qualities, it is an excellent oil for the skin, especially acne and cold sores. Bergamot is an effective deodorizer, which makes it an excellent choice for scenting a room. Bergamot essential oil blends well with almost all other oils. It is widely used in perfumery. CAUTION: Bergamot increases photosensitivity of the skin so should not be applied before exposure to direct sunlight.

Properties: Balancing, regenerative, uplifting, confidence building
Blends well with: eucalyptus, geranium, juniper, jasmine, lavender, lemon, patchouli, roman chamomile, ylang, ylang

Lemon

This essential oil is considered the "golden gift of the sun," carrying vitality into the body, mind, and soul. The lemon tree is native to Asia, although it now grows wild in the Mediterranean, particularly in Spain and Portugal. It is cultivated extensively in many parts of the world, including California. The oil was used by the ancient Egyptians as an antidote to food poisoning and to cure epidemics of fever. In most European countries it was regarded as a cure-all, but its main use was as a treatment for infectious diseases. This versatile oil is extremely effective in the diffuser to reduce the effects of mental fatigue and listlessness while regulating the body's natural immune system and resistance levels. Lemon oil eases anxiety, depression, confusion. It brings cheer and strength in times of illness and convalescence. The antiseptic qualities of lemon make it a natural alternative to synthetic household cleansers as it effectively purifies stale air, kills bacteria and freshens almost any atmosphere. In steam facials, it is useful for the treatment of acne and congested oily skin. Lemon oil aids healing of wounds and infections.
CAUTION: Avoid use 6 hours before prolonged exposure to direct sunlight.

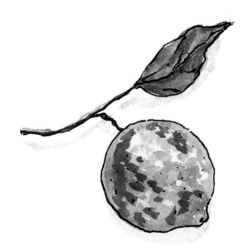

Properties: Antiseptic, antibacterial, uplifting, energizing, refreshing, strengthening
Blends well with: eucalyptus, frankincense, geranium, juniper, lavender, roman chamomile, rose, sandalwood, ylang ylang

Clary Sage

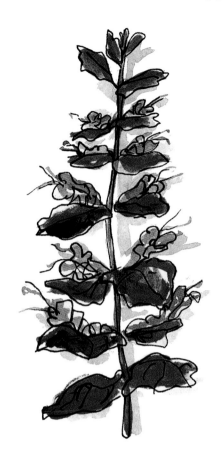

In ancient times, clary sage was highly regarded by the Greeks and Romans for its euphoric and aphrodisiac properties while the Germans favored it for its ability to intensify the intoxicating effects of Muscatel wines. This tall, biennial herb grows in most parts of the world and provides a powerful aromatic, yet benevolent, euphoric oil.

The plant is widely used as a culinary herb in soups and stews. Its oil is used in the perfume industry. The uplifting and inspiring action of clary sage creates a sense of well-being useful for times of depression and nervous tension. It is useful as an aid in adjusting to change and helping put things into perspective. Clary sage has a strong, dry, and nutty aroma. It encourages creative thought, but because it can also cause sleepiness, it is best used for times of pleasure and relaxation. For this reason, clary sage should not be used before driving or any function requiring focused concentration. This essential oil is very useful for women who suffer from PMS or menopausal symptoms. Clary sage has a place in many body care products, especially for hair since it stimulates the scalp and for skin since it is a cell regenerator. Clary sage is grown in many countries and its oil is distilled from its flowering tops and leaves. CAUTION: If used in too high a dilution, clary sage can be intoxicating. Never mix its use with alcohol consumption. Use caution when driving after exposure to clary sage. Also caution should be used with pregnant women.

Properties: Earthy, pungent, euphoric, antidepressant, calming
Blends well with: bergamot, frankincense, geranium, jasmine, juniper, lavender, sandalwood

Frankincense

This essential oil is extracted from the gum resin of the bark of the frankincense tree. Its aroma is warm, rich, and slightly lemony. Most people recognize the scent of the oil from smelling incense and remember the biblical story of the three kings offering frankincense to the baby Jesus. The use of this oil dates back more than 4000 years. Both calming and uplifting, it brings reassurance and aids meditation. Frankincense has a powerful effect in clearing lung and nasal passages and can ease shortness of breath. It is also useful for sore throats and strengthening the immune system. In skin care, the oil has an anti-inflammatory effect making it an ideal choice for mature and dry skin.

Properties: Anti-inflammatory, antidepressant, spiritual
Blends well with: bergamot, geranium, lavender, patchouli, sandalwood

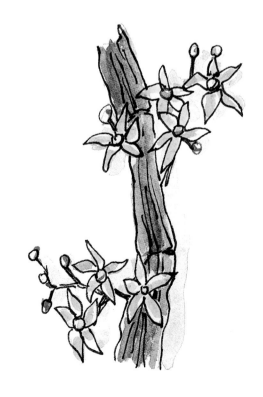

Patchouli

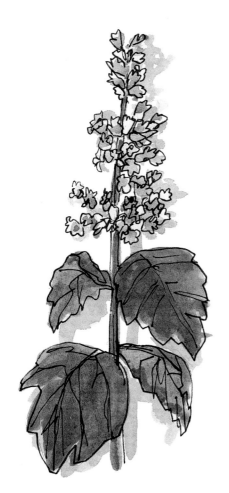

Patchouli evokes a strong response in anyone who smells this essential oil. It is either loved or hated. Its pungent, earthy scent is long-lasting and is considered an aphrodisiac. Very little of the oil is needed to create a lovely essence, massage oil, or skin care blend. Patchouli is believed to be antidepressant, anti-inflammatory, antiseptic, sedative in low doses, and stimulating in high doses. This oil helps regenerate skin cells and is useful for aged skin, cracked skin, acne, dandruff, eczema, and other skin problems. Patchouli oil has been used in combination with both sandalwood and frankincense to aid meditation and contemplation. Patchouli originated in Malaysia and India. Now it is also grown in the West Indies, China, Indonesia, and Paraguay. The essence has been widely used in perfumery as a fixative. Patchouli is a nurturing oil when someone is in a state of anxiety and depression.

Properties: Romantic, uplifting, soothing
Blends well with: bergamot, clary sage, frankincense, geranium, lavender, rose, rosewood, sandalwood

Sweet Orange

Sweet Orange is another citrus essential oil which brings the healing, rejuvenating qualities of solar energy into the body/mind system. It promotes mental clarity and emotional balance and is a wonderful oil for the doldrums of winter. Sweet orange assists in resolving and releasing deep emotional issues. This is a very inexpensive oil which can be used lavishly in the home. This oil is relaxing and calming, soothing the nerves and aiding sleep. The essence of orange comes from the fruit of the tree which originated in China, but now also grows in France, Portugal, the Americas, and the Mediterranean lands. It is a very refreshing oil, enabling one to feel awake and cheerful, while relaxed. Soothing to the nervous and digestive system, it will draw the stiffness out of sore, tense muscles when added to a massage blend. It is a good cleanser of the blood that will detoxify and rejuvenate the skin, returning to it the quality of youth. CAUTION: As with all citrus oils, use can increase photosensitivity of the skin. Do not apply before exposure to direct sunlight.

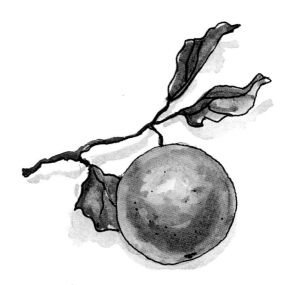

Properties: Bright, cheerful, regenerative, balancing
Blends well with: bergamot, lemon, jasmine, sandalwood, ylang ylang

Sandalwood

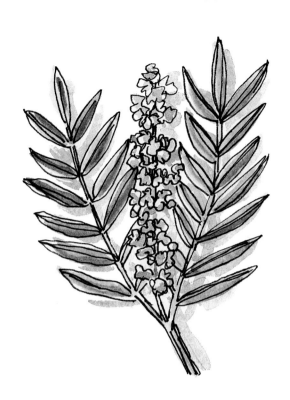

This essential oil has been used in perfumery for over 4000 years. It has been used extensively in Chinese medicine. Imported from India, it is distilled from the heartwood of the sandalwood tree, which must be at least 30 years old before it is ready for production of the oil. It has a woody, balsamic aroma. In modern times, it continues to be used in incense, perfumes and cosmetics. It is a calming oil, enhancing meditation and sleep. In skin care, sandalwood serves as a moisturizer. Its scent is long-lasting, uplifting, and is soothing to the spirit.

Properties: Antidepressant, antiseptic, meditative, aphrodisiac
Blends well with: bergamot, frankincense, geranium, jasmine, lavender, lemon, rose, ylang ylang

Ylang ylang

This essential oil is extracted from the flowers of a tree grown in Indonesia. The flowers are strewn on beds of newlyweds as a good luck/fertility wish. Ylang ylang is a soothing, calming oil which produces a sense of well-being. The oil has been credited with lowering blood pressure when the condition is caused by stress or shock. It is considered an aphrodisiac creating an exotic, erotic reaction. Because the essential oil has such a strong essence, a little goes a long way. The scent is long-lasting and is an excellent fixative in perfumes. Ylang ylang becomes more powerful when combined with other oils. In skin care products, ylang ylang is good for oily skin and also for stressed skin.

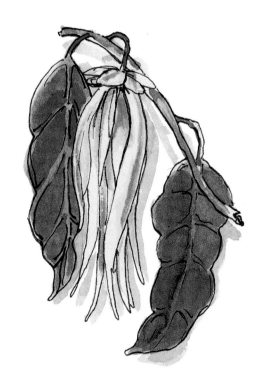

Properties: Antidepressant, aphrodisiac, euphoric, sedative
Blends well with: bergamot, jasmine, lavender, lemon, patchouli, rose, rosewood, sandalwood

The Most Expensive Essential Oils – But Worth Every Drop

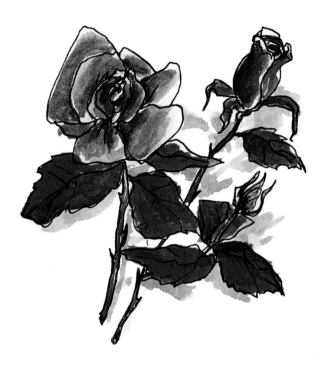

Rose Absolute or Otto

Rose is one of the most expensive oils. It is a valuable addition to your stock because of its wonderful aroma, its enhancing properties, and its synergistic complement to blends. A few drops will go a long way so even a small bottle will last for awhile. The extraction of this oil is done through a solvent extraction from the fresh petal, requiring up to 5000 pounds of petals to make 1 pound of essential oil. Rose oil is a very spiritual oil that has been used in ceremonies throughout history. The oil has many uses, among them its effectiveness in dealing with depression, grief, sadness, lost love, and low periods in one's life. Rose is an excellent oil for women to help with balancing the hormonal system and with emotional issues. It is a luxurious addition to perfumes, massage oils, and skin care products, adding a rich, rosy fragrance. It also helps broken capillaries, aids sensitive and inflamed skin, and is a wonderful tonic for mature skin.

Properties: Antidepressant, aphrodisiac, balancing, spiritual
Blends well with: bergamot, clary sage, geranium, jasmine, lavender, patchouli, Roman chamomile, sandalwood, ylang ylang

Jasmine Absolute

This deep, sweet, floral-scented essential oil comes from the white, star-shaped flowers growing on a sturdy, climbing shrub that is grown in many parts of the world. The flowers – 8000 needed to make just a single gram of oil – are picked only at night when their aroma is even more powerful. This oil is considered one of the most precious oils available. The oil earns its place among "should haves" with its many benefits: an exotic, sensuous essence; an ability to blend with just about any other essential oil; its effective use as an antidepressant, aphrodisiac, sedative, and antiseptic oil. Only a few drops of this beloved scent can do wonders for any blend. Jasmine oil can be used in skin care, especially for dry, irritated or sensitive skin and is helpful in treating muscular spasms, coughs, and hoarseness, uterine disorders, and stress-related conditions. It has been extensively used in perfumes, soaps, toiletries, and cosmetics.

Properties: Aphrodisiac, antidepressant, sedative
Blends well with: any essential oil but especially with bergamot, clary sage, geranium, rose, sandalwood, ylang ylang

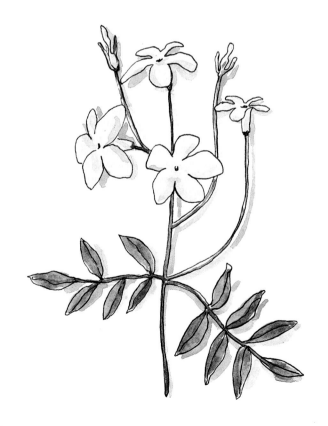

Neroli

This oil has the reputation of being one of the most precious and expensive oils available. Neroli essential oil comes from the fragrant white blossoms of the Seville orange tree, and its reputation of being such an expensive oil comes from the fact that one ton of blossoms is needed to make one pound of essential oil. Neroli provides relaxing and uplifting effects on the nervous system, easing anxiety and depression and helping with any stress-related condition. It is a rejuvenator and is therefore a useful ingredient in skin care products, especially for dry, irritated skin and for dermatitis and acne problems. It is a good oil to use for scars and stretch marks as well as for the mature skin since it tones complexion and softens wrinkles. Neroli is used in perfume as well as colognes and toilet waters. As with other expensive oils, a little will go a long way and since neroli blends well with just about any other essential oil, it is a very versatile oil.

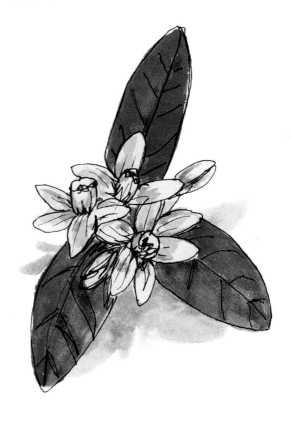

Properties: Antidepressant, rejuvenator, aphrodisiac, stimulant
Blends well with: any essential oil but especially with citrus oils such as lemon and sweet orange, chamomile, clary sage, frankincense, patchouli, rose, geranium, sandalwood, ylang ylang

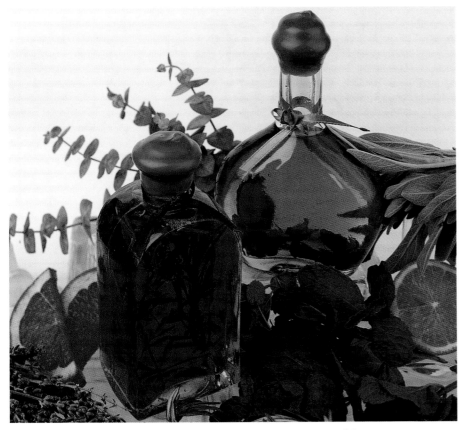

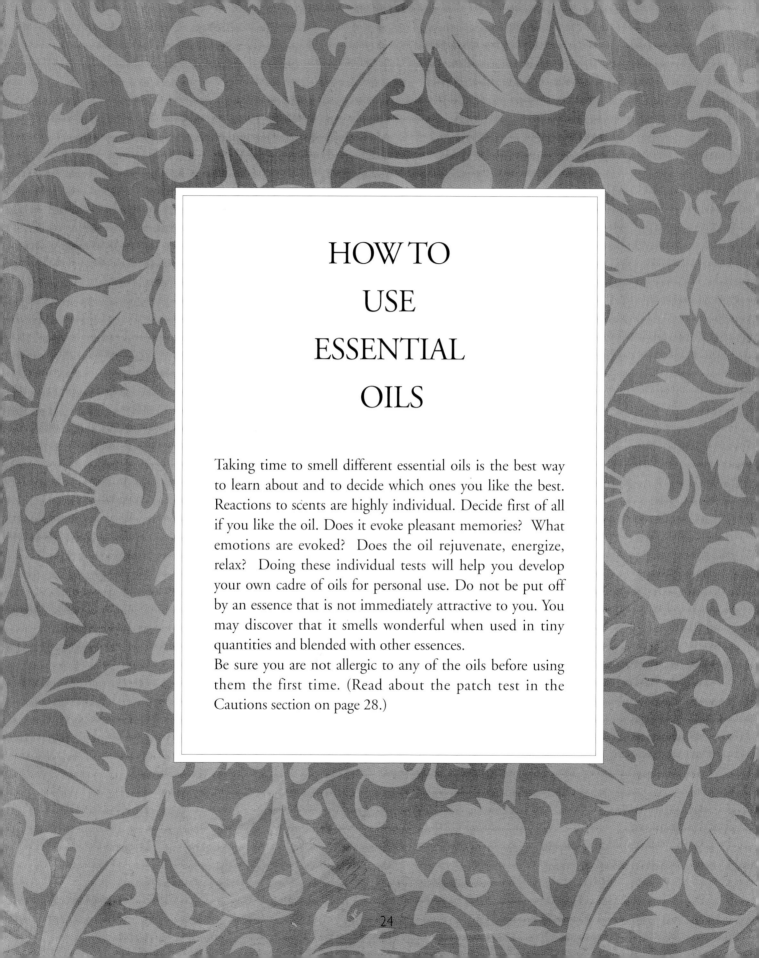

HOW TO
USE
ESSENTIAL
OILS

Taking time to smell different essential oils is the best way to learn about and to decide which ones you like the best. Reactions to scents are highly individual. Decide first of all if you like the oil. Does it evoke pleasant memories? What emotions are evoked? Does the oil rejuvenate, energize, relax? Doing these individual tests will help you develop your own cadre of oils for personal use. Do not be put off by an essence that is not immediately attractive to you. You may discover that it smells wonderful when used in tiny quantities and blended with other essences.

Be sure you are not allergic to any of the oils before using them the first time. (Read about the patch test in the Cautions section on page 28.)

Where To Find Essential Oils

Essential oils can be purchased in herb shops, health food stores, and from mail order distributors. Wherever you purchase your oils, be sure to buy from a reputable source that guarantees purity as well as quality. Essential oils vary widely in price. The distillation processes vary from oil to oil and require laboratory equipment and a large amount of materials for a small yield of oil. Some plants, like rose and jasmine, contain very little essential oil and require enormous amounts to yield even 1 oz. of oil. Therefore, beware of a display of oils with all of them the same price - they are probably synthetic blends. Make sure the oil is packaged in a dark glass bottle and is labeled "pure essential oil" - not a fragrance oil which is synthetic. Overall, the better the quality of the oil, the greater will be its therapeutic powers.

Carrier Oils: A Description

The majority of essential oils must be mixed with a carrier oil in order to be used directly on the skin. Because of their concentrated nature, the oils can irritate the skin if not diluted.

Carrier or base oils are vegetable oils used for diluting pure essential oils. They are more than just vehicles for essential oils, however, since they often have healthy benefits of their own. Combined with essential oils, they will add considerably to the dynamics of the blend as they are used in various preparations, such as bath, body, facial, and massage products as well as applying directly on the skin surface. By adding the aromatic essences to one or a combination of recommended base oils, the benefits of the essential oils are spread out over a larger area of the body and can penetrate a wider surface of skin. Since essential oils are so potent and should never be applied directly to the skin (except for a few of the oils such as lavender), their potency can be suitably diluted in carrier/base oils so as not to contact the skin directly. As a general rule, the ratio of essential oil to carrier/base oil for adults should fall between 2%-3%. This translates to about 40-60 drops

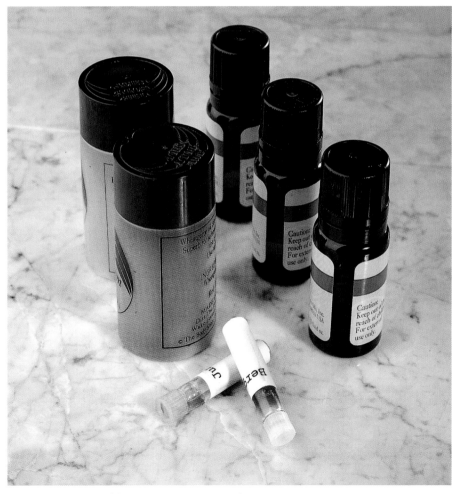

Carrier Oils: A Description (cont.)

to a 4 oz. bottle of carrier oil, 20-30 drops to a 2 oz. bottle, and 6-9 drops for a 1/2 oz. bottle.

You may choose from a variety of bases, depending on individual needs and preferences. Select a base that is as high a quality as your pure essential oil. Never use a synthetic or mineral oil base which does not penetrate the skin nor provide therapeutic aspects. Base oils are available in quantities from 1 ounce on up. Buy them in the smallest quantity available if you cannot use the oils within 3-6 months of purchase. This will help avoid oils becoming rancid. Jojoba oil, which is a wax,

is the only carrier/base oil that will not eventually oxidize and become rancid. So buy in the size you plan to use in the 3-6 month time period. Usually 1 to 4 ounces is a good amount to have on hand to start. After using them for awhile, you will discover which you prefer and can buy accordingly.

Carrier/Base oils can be obtained from health food stores, herb shops, or through mail order and should be non-refined cold-pressed oils, rather than heat-treated or refined oils. Even without the addition of essential oils, these vegetable oils are health treatments in themselves.

Carrier Oils Types

Following is a description of the carrier/base oils you may want to have on hand for experimentation. Most recipes in this book can be made with any of the carrier/base oils. Choose the one (or combination) that best suits your skin type.

Apricot kernel oil: Good for all types of skin, especially useful on sensitive and aging skin. One of the lightest oils to use. Very good for a facial oil.

Avocado oil: A nutrient-rich base oil with a high content of vitamins, protein, lecithin, and essential fatty acids. Beneficial for all skin types, but especially for mature, wrinkled, dry, and itchy skin.

Evening primrose oil: Expensive but a wonderful oil for skin care since it increases and protects skin cell

function and works as a skin rejuvenator. The oil can quickly become rancid so should be refrigerated. A small portion can be added to skin creams and lotions to increase effectiveness. It is useful for dry skin, eczema, and psoriasis.

Grapeseed oil: A nice, light, non-odoriferous oil. Makes a nice massage oil by itself or combined with sweet almond oil. Easily absorbed by the skin, suiting all skin types.

Jojoba oil: Nourishing to the skin and hair. An oil rich in Vitamin E which can be used alone or mixed with other base oils. Suitable for all skin types. Actually a wax so unlikely to become rancid (unlike most of the other vegetable oils). Contains antibacterial properties so is very good for the treatment of acne.

Sweet almond oil: Great base for massage, bath, body, and skin-care products because it is so nourishing to the skin. Contains a variety of vitamins and minerals, most notably Vitamin D. Scentless. Suitable for all skin types, especially dry or irritated skin.

Wheat germ oil: An antioxidant oil; adding a small proportion (such as 1 tablespoon to every 2 ounces of massage or body oil) to a basic mix will retain the freshness of the blend and help extend the product's shelf life. High in vitamins E, A and B as well as in mineral and protein content. Particularly beneficial to dry and mature skin. Also helps heal scar tissue, soothe burns, and smooth stretch marks.
CAUTION: This oil should not be used on people who have wheat intolerance.

Blending

Blending is a very important part of aromatherapy; it is the creative part of the process. Each essential oil has an essence of its own, but when combined with other compatible oils in a blend, the combination becomes more powerful than the sum of its parts. In other words, a synergy is created. A complex chemical is created that is more potent than any one oil used on its own and better results can be achieved without increasing the dosage. It is important to know the properties of each oil in order to achieve this blend, but some guidelines will help in your own experimentation with making your own blends.

• Blend oils with similar properties (invigorating, calming, etc.).

• Start with the blends recommended in this book. When you are ready to develop blends of your own, use no more than 3 oils until you are comfortable with the basic principles.

• Blend 1 drop at a time because even 1 drop can transform a blend.

• Write down all blends so you can repeat your successes and avoid the blends that didn't work.

• Make small quantities of blends until you're sure you will use the blend frequently.

• Aromatherapy blends will keep longer than unused carrier/base oils but still will eventually go rancid. Store properly for a shelf life of at least 6 months.

• Mix blends in glass cups, bottles, or bowls.

• Store blends in dark glass bottles, well-labeled (including ingredients, portions, etc.), dated and tightly sealed.

• Don't be afraid to experiment!

Equipment Needed for Making Products

Before beginning to prepare the products described in this book, set up a separate work space, an uncluttered area with good ventilation. Avoid hot rooms or areas with direct sunlight since essential oils can quickly evaporate.

Once you have acquired essential oils and carrier/base oils, plus the ingredients listed for each product, the rest of the equipment needed can usually be found in your kitchen. Below is a list of equipment you will need:

Glass measuring cups and bowls: for measuring and mixing ingredients.

Glass bottles (dark for massage oils and other blends) with dropper tops: for containing your mixtures. Use ones with dropper tops instead of rubber tops since the rubber will eventually break down. You may use clear glass or plastic bottles and containers to store the blends temporarily. All containers, including jars and bottles for creams, lotions, bath oils and salts, can be purchased from retail stores or mail order companies, or you can reuse previously used containers that have been sterilized.

Glass rods: for stirring. Using glass rods instead of wooden or plastic keeps the stirrer from absorbing the oils.

Mortar and pestle: for mixing oils and coloring into solid materials.

Labels: for every bottle or container, listing the ingredients, date of creation, and directions for use. Use your creativity in making the labels. For example, use rubber stamps, label-making computer software, or stickers. Some stores carry ready-made labels that are especially nice for handmade products.

Cautions

As noted in the individual descriptions of the most commonly used essential oils, one must be careful when using pure essential oils. They are highly concentrated and can burn. You may be allergic to some of the oils, especially if you have sensitive skin. Be cautious at first if you have never used essential oils before.

- Use the following patch test to make sure the oil(s) you are using will not cause an allergic reaction. Simply place a few drops of undiluted oil on the back of your wrist, cover with a bandage and leave for an hour. Check frequently to ensure that no irritation or redness has developed. If sensitization occurs, bathe the area with cold water and refrain from further use.
- When blending several recipes at one time or working with essential oils for extended periods, be careful about "sensory overload." This occurs when the essences become overpowering to your senses. Take breaks, work in a room with good circulation, and watch for signs that you've "had enough." If you start feeling jittery or irritable, or develop a headache, put the oils away for a later time.
- Some citrus oils are phototoxic, so avoid the use of lemon, lime, bergamot and orange for six hours before prolonged exposure to sunlight.
- Never use essential oils too near the eyes. Keep your hands away from the face, genitals, and mucous membranes when they have been in contact with oils.
- ALWAYS wash your hands before and after working with oils.
- Keep all essential oils out of the reach of children.
- Practice caution on working with and using essential oils while pregnant. Research the oils that are safe for pregnant women.
- Some health conditions, such as asthma, epilepsy, or high blood pressure, prevent use of some essential oils and some methods of application (such as inhalation).
- Remember essential oils are for external use only.
- Dilute, dilute, dilute. Very few essential oils can be used "neat," without dilution. Practice safe blending to avoid skin irritation.
- Store essential oils in dark, cool areas. Heat, sunlight, and oxygen will result in deterioration and reduce their therapeutic value. Use a tight-fitting cap on the bottle; do not store for long periods with eye droppers attached.
- Essential oils are flammable. Keep away from open flames.
- Do not set essential oils on furniture since they may damage the wood.

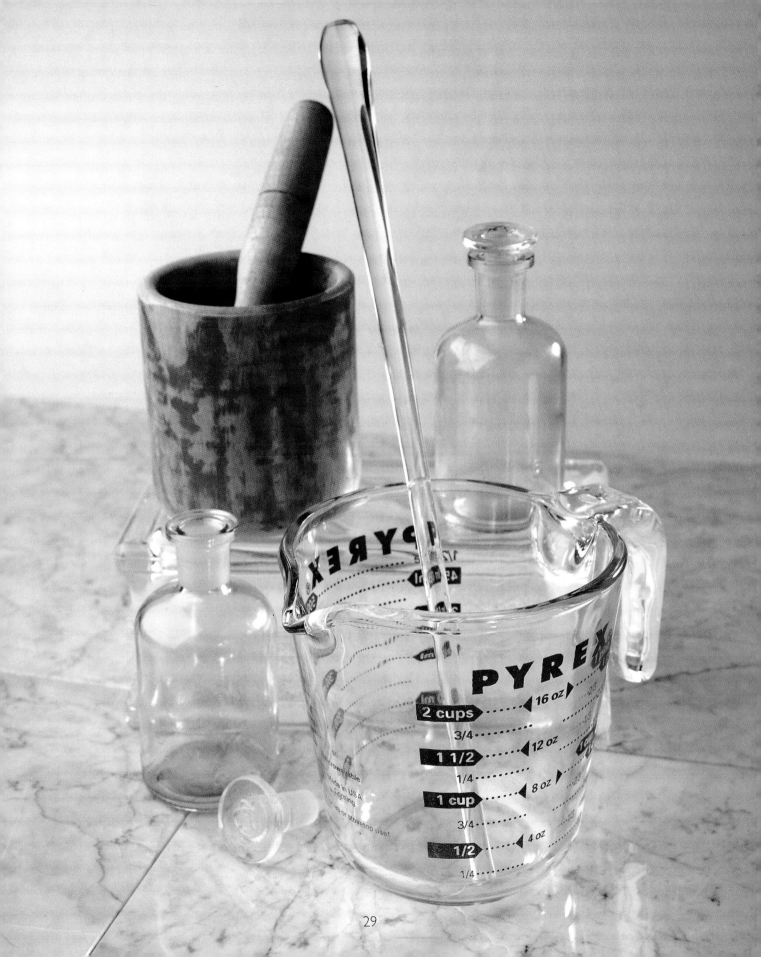

MASSAGE AS A HEALING PROCESS

Anyone can benefit from massage. Among massage's benefits are its improvement of circulation and digestion and its release of tight, sore muscles, allowing them to function properly.

RELAX

CALM

REVITALIZE

Benefits of Massage

In general, therapeutic massage releases endorphins - chemicals that affect physical well-being. One of the great advantages of massage is that it can be adapted to virtually any situation. You can do it with a partner, and it is almost as effective if you do self-massage. One of the best routes for deeper relaxation, more vitality and greater self-awareness is through massage. It is one of the most beneficial methods of using aromatherapy since it combines the healing aspect of the essential oils with the therapeutic touch of the massage.

Usually a massage oil consists of a carrier/base oil to which essential oils have been added. The carrier/base oils provide the necessary lubrication on the skin to make sure that massage strokes can be performed in a flowing manner. They also provide nutrition for the skin since they contain the fatty acids and vitamins that are vital to maintaining healthy skin.

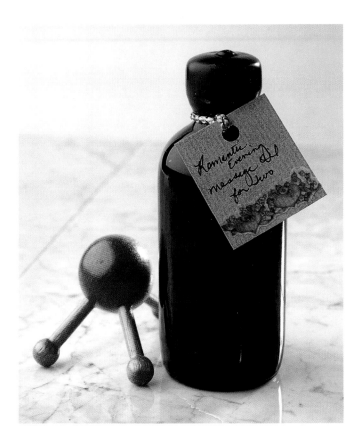

RECIPE

Romantic Evening Massage Oil

2 oz. sweet almond oil (or any appropriate base oil)

10 drops ylang ylang

10 drops jasmine

5 drops sandalwood

5 drops patchouli

Blend well and bottle.

Self-Massage

Although it is not possible to do a complete body massage by using self-massage, and therapeutically, it cannot equal the experience of being massaged by someone else, you will find that there are many times when you can help relieve your body of tense, aching, tired muscles by using a few, simple techniques. Not only does self-massage help the physical system, but it also gives you a psychological boost when stressed or tired.

Many activities inevitably lead to tensions in one part of the body or another, and regular quick massages can help to ease these tensions and to prevent more chronic aches and pains, or even injury. At any time of the day, a short self-massage can help you to feel revitalized and full of energy. It will reduce the impact of stresses, both physical and mental. A firm massage will be invigorating; a slower, gentle massage will be relaxing.

In this chapter I will give you some self-massage techniques to start using. All massage should be done with the flow of the body, in other words, toward the heart. For example, when working with the feet, work from the toes to the heel.

Recipes for complementary blends will follow each technique. NOTE: Massage oil mixtures can be blended in advance and kept on hand in dark, glass bottles in a cool, dark place. Do not prepare them more than 2 months in advance. A good general base/carrier oil to use is sweet almond oil or choose one especially good for your skin type, e.g., grapeseed oil for oily skins. For a full body massage, 4 teaspoons of massage oil is usually adequate; for the face, 2 teaspoons is enough. For a general rule of thumb, use 10 drops of essential oil per 4 teaspoons carrier oil and 5 drops per 2 teaspoons carrier oil.

❦ GETTING STARTED

Prepare your aromatherapy blend to suit your needs then, if possible, take a bath or shower. The oils penetrate more readily when the skin is warm and slightly damp. You may even do some of the self-massage techniques while in the bath, especially massage for tense muscles and for tired feet.

❦ SETTING THE MOOD

Before beginning your self-massage, find a quiet, warm area. Minimize distractions by closing the door, letting others know you do not wish to be disturbed, turning the phone and answer machine off. Light one or more candles, if you wish, adding complementary essential oil to the melted wax. Some people enjoy music; others enjoy the quiet time. Prepare your massage blend; you may keep the blend in the bottle and just pour on to the hands as needed or use a glass bowl to hold the blend. In either case, always warm the oil in your hands before applying to the body. Erase negative thoughts from your mind, and enjoy this time of renewal and rejuvenation. It may help to begin the massage with a bit of deep breathing to begin the relaxation of the body, then be sure to breathe evenly throughout the massage.

❦ MASSAGE TERMS TO KNOW

The defined terms that follow are used both in massage and self-massage. The movements are easily mastered.

- **Stroking (Effleurage):** This movement is used most frequently in massage because it is the first and main stroke of massage. It helps warm the muscles of the body and helps it to relax. The movement is free-flowing and continuous, made with the hand(s) staying flat and using steady pressure. Strokes can be applied with light to medium pressure with the whole hand making contact with the body. Allow the hands to remain relaxed and supple as they mold to the contours of the body. The object is to allow the strokes to flow across the body. Apply firmer pressure as you move toward the heart and lighten the pressure as you move away from the heart. Be sure to keep enough oil on your hands to allow them to glide along the body surface.
- **Kneading:** This technique relaxes deeper muscles, improving blood circulation and bringing in fresh blood while eliminating toxins. It is best used on the muscular and fleshy parts of the body, e.g., the tops of shoulders, waist, buttocks, thighs, calves. Perform this technique by gripping the part of the body that is tense and use a squeezing motion to loosen the tension. A lighter kneading movement can be used in less fleshy parts of the body, such as the tops of arms. Kneading movements should be followed by stroking in order to soothe the area and boost circulation.
- **Thumb pressure:** This movement is used to ease tension and relax the body. It is performed by using the thumbs to apply gentle pressure on tense parts of the body, e.g., the feet, or along the spine.
- **Static pressure:** This movement works well on tension areas in the neck and shoulders, soles of feet, and spine. No oil is actually needed for this movement. Use the pads of the thumbs to press into the skin firmly. Hold for up to 10 seconds. Release slowly then move to any other areas of tension. Do not gouge the skin - never poke sharply.

Tense Neck

Aching, tense muscles are most frequently experienced in the neck and shoulders. This is the area of the body most inclined to gather the tension from everyday stress, emotional upset or bad posture. As you get tired, your posture tends to droop and the rounded shapes makes your shoulders and neck ache even more. Release mounting tension before your shoulders become permanently hunched up around your ears. If the tensions are not released, you will be more likely to have contracted muscles restricting the blood flow to the head and brain. This usually brings on a headache, making you feel tired and irritable.

1. Shrug your shoulders, lifting them up as far as possible and then letting them drop down and relax completely.
2. Place some massage oil into the palm of one of your hands, warm it by rubbing both hands together, then spread it with flowing strokes over the upper back and neck and across the shoulders and tops of the arms.
3. Knead your neck and shoulders by firmly gripping your opposite shoulder with your hand and use a squeezing motion to loosen the tension. Move slowly along the shoulder, squeezing firmly several times. Repeat on the other side, using the opposite hand. This will help restore oxygenated blood into the neck and shoulders thereby relieving tension.
4. Grip the back of the neck with the fingers of both hands and squeeze. Use thumb pressure to relax the muscles leading up either side of the neck. Work up as far as the base of the skull and down again to the shoulders. Repeat several times until the tension begins to be released.
5. Shrug the shoulders again. Take a deep breath and relax the shoulders.

Preventive Measures: Work on improving your posture. Stand and sit erect. Notice that when you are tired, you allow your body to droop and sag. Help prevent the accompanying tired and achy muscles by reminding yourself to relax the shoulders, keeping the head and neck in line with the spine.

RECIPES

Massage Blend for Tense Neck

Recipe #1

- To 1 oz. of carrier/base oil (use appropriate oil for your skin type), add 8 drops lavender, 4 drops lemon, and 3 drops Roman chamomile or peppermint (2% dilution) oils.
- Store in glass bottle, preferably dark for stored blends. Clear bottles may be used if the oil will not be stored more than 2 weeks.
- Other oils that may be used as substitutes: clary sage, juniper, eucalyptus, orange, rosemary.

Recipe #2

- To 1 tablespoon of base oil, add 2 drops clary sage, 2 drops ylang ylang, and 4 drops sandalwood.

Daily Face and Neck Massage

A self-massage on the face and neck in the morning will refresh you for the day ahead and, at night, will ease away tension and the effects of stress. The rhythmic stroking of your fingertips over these areas of your body will enliven your skin, drawing the blood circulation close to its surface to nourish tissues and cells. Facial skin is delicate so work gently using a blend that suits your skin type (see page 47). NOTE: Before using massage oils on the face, remove contact lenses or eyeglasses.

1. With clean hands, pour a small amount of the massage oil into your palm and warm it between your hands. Dab the oil under your eyes with your middle fingers and allow the oil to soak in without massaging so the delicate tissues are not disturbed. Smooth the oil over the rest of your face and front and back of the neck with soft and flowing movements from your palms and fingers. This motion will begin to warm the muscles and tissues that lay beneath them.

2. Begin to stimulate the skin and ease away tension by stroking. Start with your brow and temples. Then move the fingertips of both hands over the forehead, moving from the center to the sides of your head. Use a stroking motion with your fingers as you work around both temples to clear and ease your mind. Press and squeeze along the rims of both ears with your thumbs and index finger, and then stroke behind the ears. Move both hands in a soft, counter-clockwise motion over your cheeks, then press deeply with fingertip circles over the cheeks and jaw.

3. Tap the fingertips of both hands rhythmically all over the face, starting on the forehead and then moving them over the temples, cheekbones, cheeks, jaw, and chin. This will tone the skin and stimulate circulation.

4. As a final massage step, rhythmically tap below your chin and jaw with the back of one hand.

5. To further revitalize yourself, wipe the excess oil from your hands and continue tapping all over your scalp.

6. Take a deep breath and enjoy the overall sensation you feel.

RECIPES

Deeply Moisturizing Massage Oil for the Face and Neck

Oily Skin: Add 2 drops bergamot, 1 drop lemon or geranium to 2 teaspoons grapeseed oil.

Sensitive Skin: Add 2 drops chamomile and 1 drop lavender to 2 teaspoons sweet almond oil.

Dry Skin: Add 2 drops neroli, 1 drop of frankincense, 1 drop of geranium to 1 teaspoon each of sweet almond oil and jojoba.

Quick Partial Face Massages for Overactive Mind

Use the first two fingers of both hands to gently massage the temples in a counter clockwise direction. This can also be used to deal with headaches.

Recipe: Add 2 drops of lavender and 1 drop chamomile to 1 teaspoon of carrier/base oil. If preferred, lavender oil can be used neat on the fingertips and massaged directly onto the skin.

RECIPES

Massage for Congestion/ Blocked Sinuses

Press thumbs gently into hollows of inner edge of the eyebrow. Press along the eyebrow, continuing along the bone under the eye itself. Next, press up into the sinus cavities under the ridge of the cheekbones, starting at the edge of the nose and working to the side of the face.

Recipe: Good oils to use in a blend for this massage are eucalyptus, peppermint, rosemary; 3 drops per teaspoon of carrier/base oil.

Massage to Ensure a Good Night's Sleep

Bedtime massage: Add 3 drops sandalwood, 2 drops lavender, and 2 drops chamomile to 2 teaspoons of sweet almond oil. Work into shoulders, forehead, and temples. Then drift off to sleep!

Foot Massage
THRILL YOUR TOES

The feet are generally the most neglected part of the body in terms of regular care. Yet a little care will go a long way toward helping your whole body feel more energetic and refreshed. Only a few minutes of massage will remove tension from the muscles and tendons while bringing greater relaxation to the whole body posture as stress dissolves away. If you have time, give yourself a hot, scented footbath first which will soften the skin so that it absorbs the oil more easily.

1. Begin the foot massage by pouring a small amount of the massage oil into the palm of your hand then rubbing your hands together to warm the oil. Sit comfortably, laying the calf of one leg over the thigh of the other to have good access to both sides of your foot. Cradle the foot between both hands for a minute or so to give it warmth. Spread the oil over the entire foot with flowing strokes.

2. Starting with the little toe and working toward the big toe, clasp the toe between your thumb and index finger and circle it three times to the right and then to the left. Then gently rub and squeeze each toe, including the nail tip, with the thumb and index finger. Pull each toe by gripping firmly between thumb and finger and stretch gently.

3. Make a fist with your hand and place the knuckles just above the heel of the foot. Firmly move the knuckles along the sole of the foot toward the toes. Follow with gentle strokes over the sole of the foot.

4. Move toward the ankle. Place your thumbs on the front of the ankle and use a static press to relax the ligaments and joints.

5. To finish, cradle the foot in both hands and rub briskly across the sole and instep to create heat and vitality. Hold the foot gently for a few moments before repeating the massage on the other foot.

6. After both feet have been massaged, put your hands over the soles of both feet to bring a sense of balance to the body. Take a deep breath and enjoy the revitalization of the entire body.

RECIPE

Foot Massage

Tired Feet: Add 3 drops lavender, 1 drop peppermint to 2 teaspoons sweet almond oil.

Swollen Feet: Add 3 drops lavender, 2 drops chamomile to 2 teaspoons sweet almond oil.

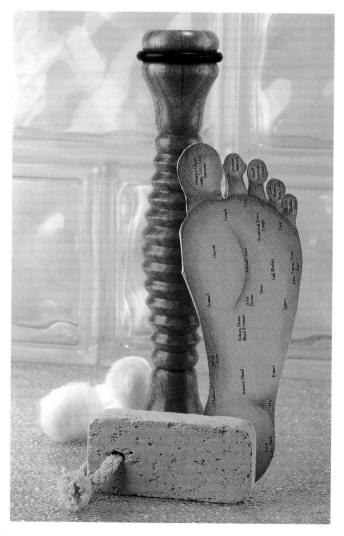

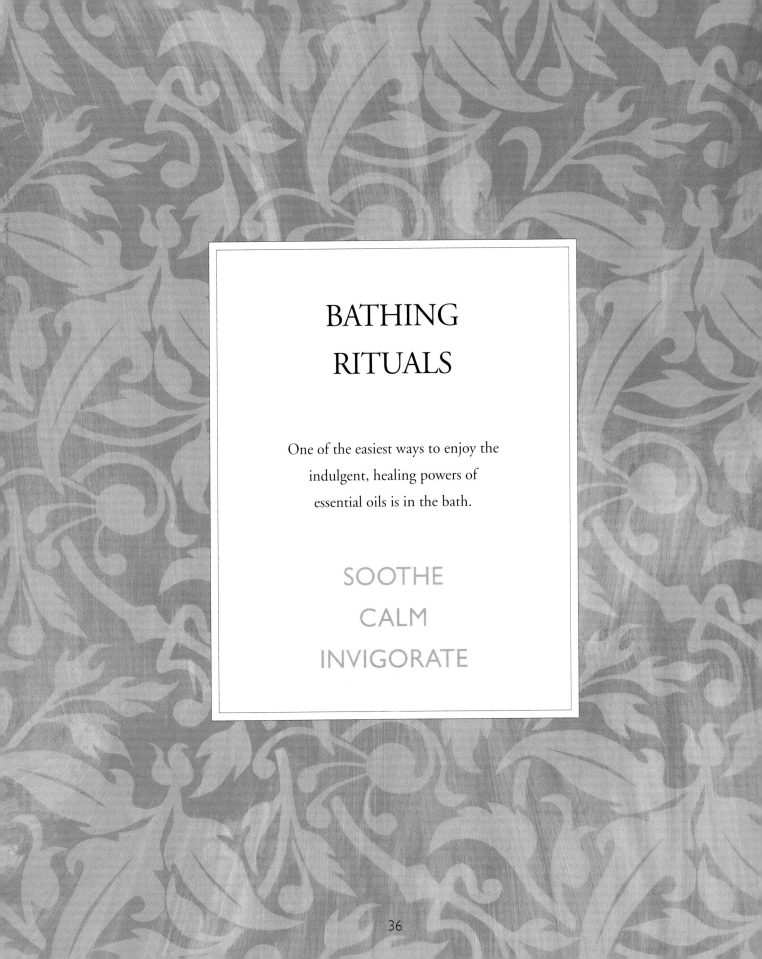

BATHING
RITUALS

One of the easiest ways to enjoy the
indulgent, healing powers of
essential oils is in the bath.

SOOTHE

CALM

INVIGORATE

Benefits of Bathing Rituals

Essential oils and baths have synergistic effects. They enhance the ability of the other to soothe, calm, or invigorate the body by allowing you to both breathe the wonderful aromas as well as absorbing them through the skin. The oils can be used pure, using 5-10 drops depending on the strength of the oil (for example, eucalyptus and peppermint would have a maximum of 5 drops, but up to 10 drops could be used with the milder lavender). Put the oils into the bath just before getting in. If added to the water while the tub is filling, much of the oils' essences will go up in the steam and very little will be left to be absorbed by the skin. If using the essences "neat" (without dilution), be sure to swirl them in the water before stepping in to avoid any possible skin irritations that might occur with direct skin contact. This method of using essential oils in the bath is good to use when you will be washing your hair and would not want the oily appearance that an oil blend would leave.

Since essential oils are not water soluble and do not fully disperse when added directly to bath water, diluting the oils is another effective way to use them. Essential oils may be diluted in unscented liquid soap for a bubble bath effect, combined with bath salts, or mixed with base/carrier oils in a blend or as a bath oil or body scrub. The combinations are numerous, but the results are the same: bathing is a luxury you shouldn't be without.

Remember that the temperature of the water can also be used to complement the effect of the oils. For example, for a refreshing, stimulating bath, use cool water with rosemary or peppermint. For a restful sleep, use warm water with lavender or chamomile to soothe the jagged edges. Avoid hot baths - your skin will perspire and be less able to absorb the essential oils. Also, hot water dehydrates the skin and causes the essential oils to evaporate much more quickly. A warm or cool bath allows the oils to envelop your body delightfully when you slip into your bath and will penetrate your skin and diffuse into the tissues. Breathe deeply, relax, and enjoy this time of quiet – but necessary – indulgence.

RECIPES

Try the following oils by themselves or diluted with carrier/base oils (2-5 drops of essential oil per teaspoon of carrier/base oil or 6-15 drops essential oil per table-spoon of carrier/base oil).

For calming baths (evening): lavender, chamomile, sweet orange

For stimulating baths (morning): lemon, rosemary, peppermint

For baths to relieve muscular aches and rheumatic pains: juniper, rosemary, lemon, eucalyptus

For baths to relieve cold and flu symptoms: eucalyptus, lavender, peppermint

For baths to relieve symptoms of PMS: clary sage, lavender, bergamot

Bath Oil

Bath oil is not only beautiful to look at but can be used for massage and in the bath as well. High quality bath oils can be quite expensive to buy but can be made at a fraction of the cost. They are very easy to make but look extravagant! Bath oils are a great treatment for dry skin and especially healing in the winter months. They make great gifts for someone who has a very stressful life and needs to unwind with a long, luxurious bath.

Supplies needed:
Carrier Oils: such as sweet almond oil, avocado, jojoba, apricot kernel, wheat germ oil, or grapeseed oil (you may use a combination of oils as well)
Essential oils
Dried herbs: (optional) They do make the oil look pretty but are not necessary for creating a beautiful bath oil.
Pretty bottles in various sizes and shapes
Funnel
Corks
Ribbon or raffia
Sealing wax
Labels

Tips:
Decorate the neck of the bottle with raffia or ribbon (if you have not used either in the process of sealing the bottle top).

Add a few sprigs of dried flowers, if desired. Label the bottle or provide a card with the bottle that gives the ingredients and directions for use. Usually 2-3 tablespoons of bath oil per bath is sufficient to receive the benefits of the oil.

CAUTION: Be careful with using bath oils in Jacuzzis. If you own a Jacuzzi or you're giving the oil to someone who does, use the Dispersing Bath Oil recipe.

❧ BASIC BATH OIL RECIPE

This recipe makes 16 oz. and can be used for a single bottle or several smaller ones. A separate container is always used for the blending before placing in sterilized, clean containers.

16 oz. of base oil*
24 - 30 drops of essential oil
8 vitamin E capsules**

Blend the oils - base oils first, then essential oils - in a sterile container. Break open the vitamin E capsules, emptying them into the oil and stirring or shaking well. You may insert dried flowers or other decorations into the decorative bottle (clean and sterilized) before filling with the oil mixture. Insert the cork top and seal the bottle top with sealing wax.

RECIPES

Soothing Bath Oil
To the Basic Bath Oil Recipe, add:
20 drops of lavender essential oil
10 drops of geranium essential oil

Dried lavender flower stems and rose petals/buds may be inserted in the oil if desired.

Stimulating Bath Oil
To the Basic Bath Oil Recipe, add:
20 drops of rosemary essential oil
10 drops of juniper essential oil

Add dried flowers if desired.

RECIPES

Winter Blahs Bath Oil
To Basic Bath Oil Recipe, add:
20 drops sweet orange essential oil
10 drops geranium essential oil

Orange slices or rind may be inserted in the oil if desired.

Floral Garden Bath Oil
To Basic Bath Oil Recipe, add:
12 drops rose absolute, rosewood or geranium essential oil
8 drops ylang ylang essential oil
8 drops lavender essential oil
2 drops patchouli essential oil

Dried flowers may be inserted in the oil if desired.

*Any combination of oils can make up the base oil. If adding wheat germ oil, delete vitamin E capsules.

**NOTE: Vitamin E acts as a preservative when added to other oils and prevents rancidity. It is excellent for all skin types and is reported to slow the aging process.

❧ DISPERSING BATH OIL

To make a bath oil that will totally disperse in the bath water, the carrier oil used must be **turkey red oil**, or sulfated castor oil. It softens water without leaving a residue on your body or the tub, making it perfect to use in a Jacuzzi. Just substitute the turkey red oil for the base oil called for in any of the above recipes. NOTE: This oil is not clear so it doesn't make as pretty an oil to use in a clear bottle as sweet almond, for example. I normally use a colored bottle for this oil so the color of the oil is disguised.

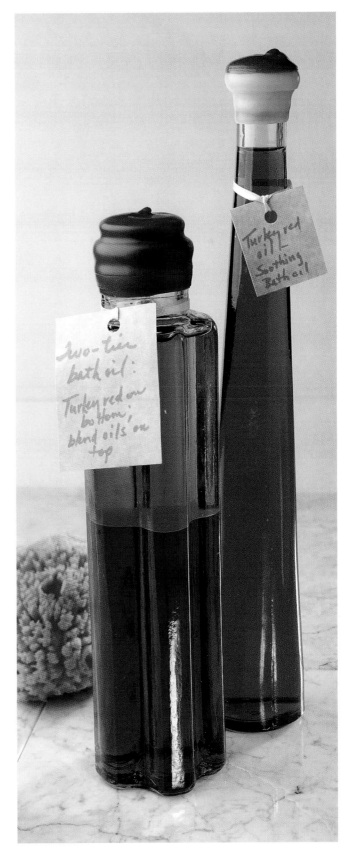

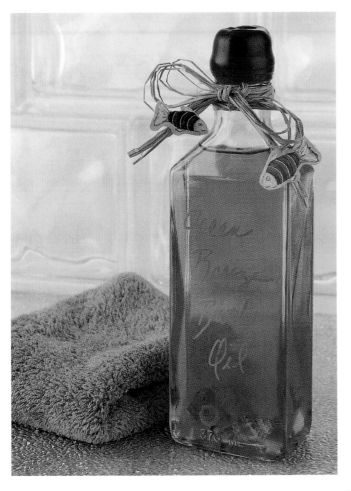

Herbal Bath Salts

Bath salts are easy to make, inexpensive, and make wonderful gifts. You can use decorative tins or jars with tight-fitting lids to hold the salts. Apothecary jars do nicely as containers for bath salts. (Tip: use a small, muslin bag of rice in the bottom of the container to absorb any moisture that might get into the container.) When properly sealed and stored, bath salts can last a long time.

Sea salt is an excellent choice for your bath salts. It detoxifies the body and conditions the water and skin. With the addition of essential oils to the salt, you have a wonderful combination. Only a small amount of essential oils is needed to make a fragrant blend.

Baking soda is also considered a salt and when added to the blend, provides another element for soothing aching muscles. It absorbs the essential oils easily and releases the scent when dissolved in bath water.

There are countless blends to use for bath salts. A basic recipe follows. It may be easily doubled.

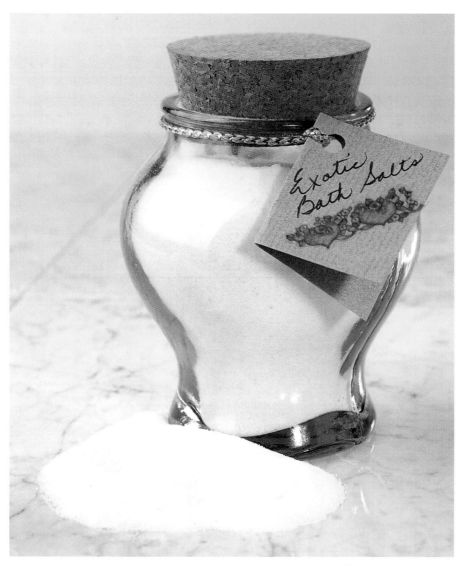

❧ BASIC SALTS RECIPE

1 cup baking soda
1 cup sea salt
10-15 drops essential oil
Few drops of food coloring, if desired

Blend together and use immediately or store in a tightly sealed container. One-fourth cup of the salts is enough for each bath.

NOTE: Add the food coloring separately to a small amount of the salts. Blend well then mix with rest of salts until desired color is visible.

TIP: If using one of the more aromatic or expensive oils, you can create a fragrant blend by using less. For example, 2-4 drops of the exotic jasmine or rose absolute when mixed thoroughly will make a very pleasant blend. Some of the stronger scents – such as eucalyptus, patchouli, peppermint, for example, may only require 6-8 drops.

RECIPES

Exotic Bath Salts

To Basic Salts Recipe, add:

5 drops jasmine absolute essential oil
3 drops rose absolute essential oil
5 drops ylang ylang essential oil

Blend thoroughly and place in appropriate container.

Relaxation Bath Salts

To Basic Salts Recipe, add:

8 drops lavender essential oil
5 drops sweet orange essential oil
Few drops blue food coloring to half the salt.

Blend food coloring in half the salt. Add essential oils to other half and blend well. Add blue salts and mix just enough for all the salt to absorb the scent but not enough to blend colors. Effect will be dappled.

Achy Joints Bath Salts

To Basic Salts Recipe, add:

4 drops eucalyptus essential oil
6 drops lavender essential oil
4 drops rosemary essential oil

Blend thoroughly and place in appropriate container.

Basic Salts Recipe (cont.)

Experiment, starting with a few drops, and increasing incrementally by a drop until you have the blend that satisfies you. REMEMBER - more is not necessarily better with essential oils. Let the mixture "mellow" a bit to see if the fragrance is strong enough before adding more.

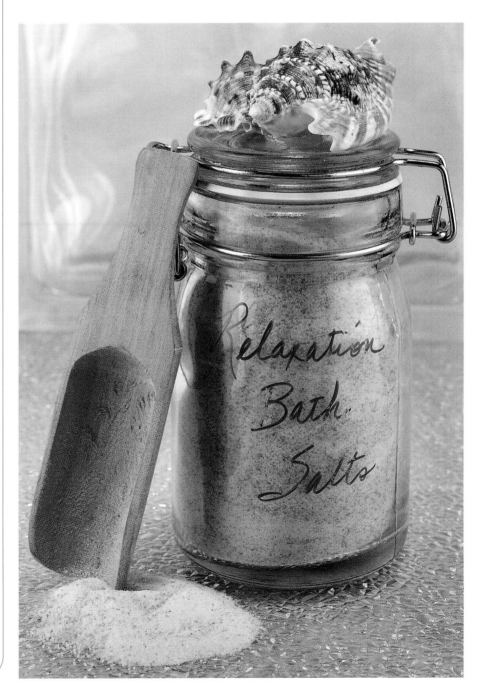

Rejuvenating Body Scrub

Another wonderful way to use sea salt with essential oils is to blend them with a base oil to make an exhilarating exfoliator. Especially good carrier oils to use for this are sweet almond, apricot kernel, or grapeseed.

To apply, stand in a bathtub or shower stall and massage the body scrub gently over the body. It is best to start with the feet and work up. Massage every part of the body except for the face and neck (too delicate); also go gently on breasts. Don't worry if a lot of the salt falls to the floor of the stall or tub; just pick up and keep using. After you have finished the massage, shower or run a warm bath and wash the salts away. Your body will be invigorated and will have a lovely scent. This is a wonderful exercise for exfoliating the entire body before bathing. After bathing, lavish your body with soothing, fragrant lotion or cream.

RECIPE

Body Scrub

2 cups sea salt
6-8 drops of essential oil blended with 1 oz. of base/carrier oil

Just combine all the ingredients together in a bowl, and mix well. Make sure all oil is thoroughly absorbed by the salt.

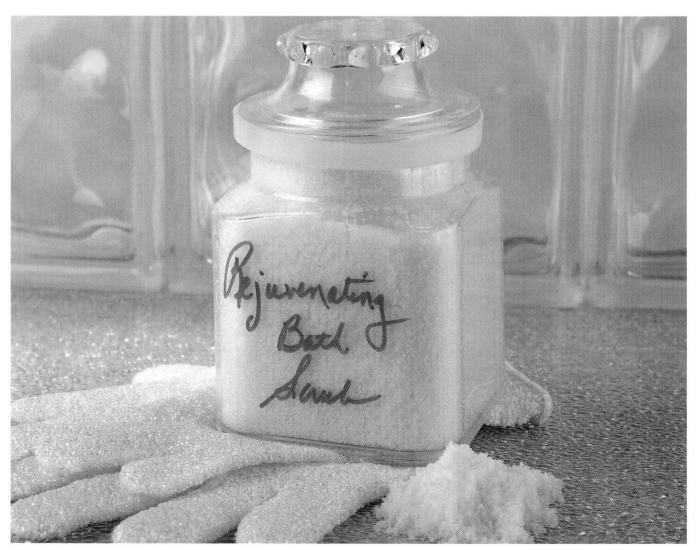

Bath Fizzies

A fun way to use bath salts in your bath is to make bath fizzies. These unique, sculpted salts are delightful as gifts and can be made in any number of shapes and sizes. The solid bath fizzy acts as a giant effervescent tablet in the bath, creating lots of bubbles, and releasing its fragrance as it dissolves. The bigger the molded fizzy, the longer it lasts. Try an assortment of sizes, shapes, colors, and fragrances. These will be a hit as a part of any gift you give.

RECIPE
Fragrant Bath Fizzies
1 cup baking soda
1/2 cup cornstarch
1/2 cup citric acid
15 drops essential oil
food color, 10 drops (optional)

Mix all ingredients in a bowl. Add food coloring to a small amount of the mix in a separate bowl. Add colored mix to remaining mix and blend. Mist the salts with a mister enough so that they hold together but not enough to start fizzing. Pack these salts into a soap mold. Flip over onto a piece of waxed paper and allow molded fizzie to dry overnight.

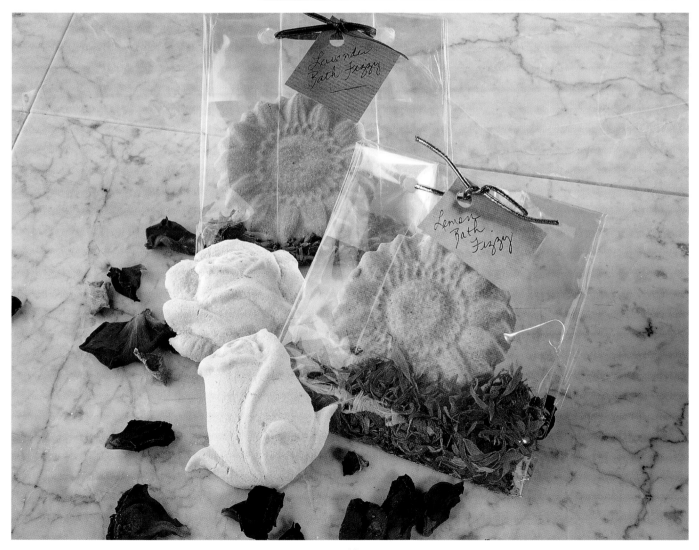

Scented Bath Vinegars

Apple cider vinegar is always a healthy addition to the bath. It is soothing, relieves dry, itchy skin, and restores natural pH to the skin. A wonderfully scented vinegar is even more pleasant to use - it provides the healthy benefits of apple cider vinegar plus the additional therapeutic properties of essential oils. Try this recipe for yourself - bottle it up in a pretty bottle and give it as a gift. It's an addictive addition to the bath!

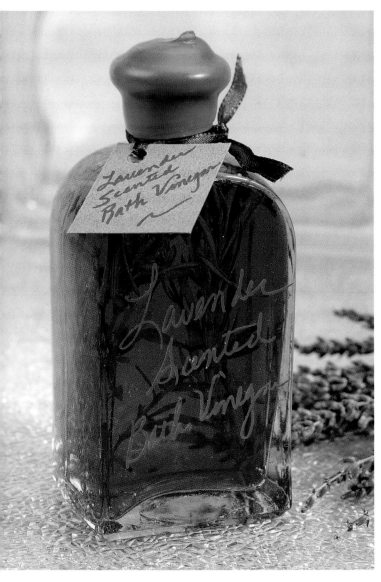

RECIPE

Scented Bath Vinegar

4 cups of apple cider vinegar
2 cups of petals of rose, lavender, lemon verbena, peppermint, or calendula
4 cups distilled water
10 drops of complementary essential oil
(according to the herb used, e.g., lavender essential oil if the lavender herb was used for the steeping material).

Steep petals in vinegar for 6-8 weeks. (To shorten this time to 2 weeks, heat the vinegar before adding the herbs.) After the steeping time, strain the mixture. I use a coffee filter in an old coffee maker holder and place on top of a container to drain. Add an equal amount of distilled water, and complementary essential oil Allow mixture to blend for a few days then pour into pretty glass bottles. You may use corked bottles and seal the cork with sealing wax as you do with bath oils.

Use 1 cup in the bath water, pouring it in as the water fills the tub. The scented vinegar also makes a good compress when you soak a wash cloth in the liquid, wring it out and apply it to the desired body area. These make unusual - but much appreciated – gifts.

After the Bath

After you've had a nice warm bath or shower, a nice way to moisturize the whole body is to use a body cream (page 51) or just use one of the base/carrier oils, such as sweet almond oil or jojoba oil, while your body is still wet. The cream or oil blends with the water left on the body and holds in the moisture. This is especially lovely in the evening when you can go to bed shortly after and let the creams and oils work on making your skin soft and fragrant while you sleep.

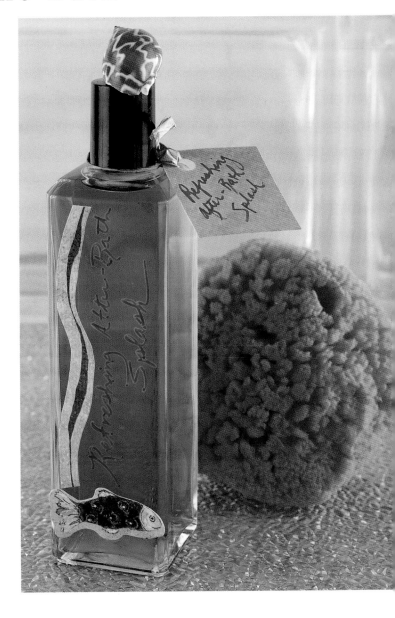

RECIPE

Refreshing After-Bath Splash

(If you are dressing to go out after your bath or shower, an after-bath splash lightly scents and refreshes the body. Use this splash also as a light cologne.)

1/2 cup distilled water
1/4 cup vodka
15 drops lavender essential oil
4 drops sandalwood essential oil

Combine together in a glass bottle (spritzer) and shake until well mixed.

❧ COMPLEMENTARY ACCESSORIES

There are many wonderful accessories for the bath available today. They add tremendously to the pleasure of bathing. Try an inflatable terry cloth bath pillow - easy to use and takes up minimal storage space when deflated. Use various scrubbies, back brushes, eye masks, and candles to make the bath a special experience. Even if you have only 20-30 minutes, a bath can make a significant difference in how you feel. Take the time for the physical and emotional benefits of baths. You may get hooked!

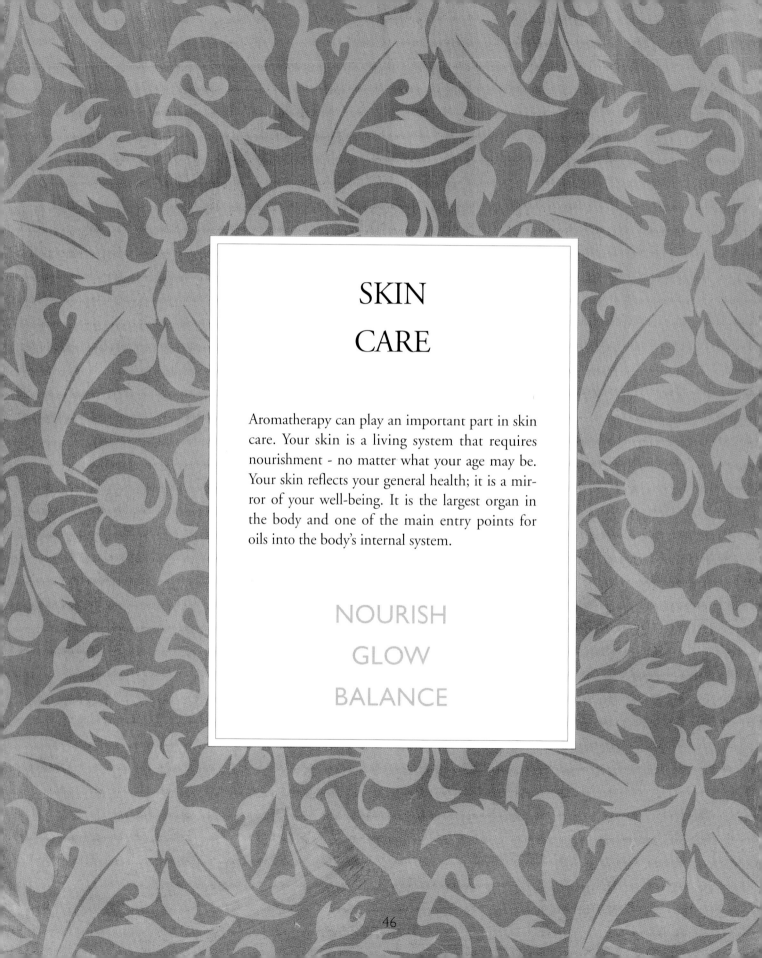

SKIN CARE

Aromatherapy can play an important part in skin care. Your skin is a living system that requires nourishment - no matter what your age may be. Your skin reflects your general health; it is a mirror of your well-being. It is the largest organ in the body and one of the main entry points for oils into the body's internal system.

NOURISH

GLOW

BALANCE

Benefits of Skin Care Products

Using essential oils in natural personal care products will be a forward step in helping your skin to glow, to radiate from the benefits of the aroma and the nourishing qualities of oils. Combined with a balanced diet, plenty of water, and exercise, many kinds of skin problems can be helped by aromatherapy.

In this chapter, I will include recipes and blends for the face, hands, feet, and entire body. Whether you are making these for yourself or for gifts, you will benefit from the aromas of the oils just by making them.

Skin Types

Dry Skin: Usually delicately textured and feels tight. Not enough oil produced naturally to keep the skin soft and supple so it is more prone to broken capillaries, flaking, and wrinkles.

Oily Skin: Tends to look greasy and have an unrefined texture due to overactive oil glands. Skin picks up dirt easily which translates into clogged pores producing blackheads and pimples.

Combination Skin: Dry areas around cheeks, neck, eyes and an oily area on the forehead, nose, and chin (T-shape).

Sensitive Skin: Can be any type but reacts to harsh products and/or rough handling.

Mature Skin: More susceptible to signs of aging - wrinkles, dryness, blotching.

Normal Skin: No such thing (except for children)! But those that approximate it have skin that is neither dry nor oily, firm and solid, finely textured with no visible spots or blemishes, soft and velvety to the touch, and unwrinkled.

Oils For Particular Skin Types or Problems

Skin-rejuvenating oils: chamomile, clary sage, eucalyptus, frankincense, geranium, jasmine, lavender, lemon, neroli, sweet orange, rose, rosemary, sandalwood, tea tree, and ylang ylang. All these oils work well on mature and dry skin.

Oily Skin: bergamot, geranium, jasmine, juniper, lavender, lemon, patchouli, rosemary, rosewood, sandalwood, clary sage, tea tree, and ylang ylang.

Dry and sensitive skin: Chamomile, frankincense, geranium, jasmine, lavender, rosewood and sandalwood.

Irritated and inflamed skin: chamomile, jasmine, lavender, patchouli, rose, clary sage, and tea tree.

Combination skin: use oils that work well with oily skin in the T-shaped zone and oils that work well with dry skin on the other parts of the face.

Face Tonics

A number of essential oils are especially good for the face. For example, lavender is good for normal, oily, combination skin types and is also beneficial for blemished, inflamed, and sensitive skin. Geranium, although not appropriate for blemished skin, does attend to the rest of the above conditions plus it's very good for dry skin. Clary sage is the mature skin's friend, helping rejuvenate cells for a more radiant complexion.

Tonics stimulate the circulation, help to reduce oiliness in the skin and help to even out skin texture. Apply after you have washed your face to help remove any residues of makeup. Always shake tonics before using since the oils will often separate from the base ingredient. Tonics can be stored in bottles, but cotton balls may also be soaked with the tonic and placed in plastic bags for instant freshening while traveling.

RECIPES

Problem Skin Relief

Dry Skin Tonic: To 3 ounces of rosewater (see recipe below) add 1 drop of sandalwood and 1 drop of rosewood.

Oily Skin Tonic: To 3 ounces of orange flower water* add 1 drop of sweet orange and 1 drop of neroli.

Acne Tonic: To 3 ounces of lavender water (see recipe below) add 1 drop of lavender and 1 drop of geranium, tea tree, or juniper.

Orange flower water can be made at home following the Rosewater Recipe but orange flowers are harder to find. Check herb shops, health food stores and catalogs that carry essential oils and other aromatherapy items to locate ready-made orange flower water.

Rosewater

2 cups distilled water
1/4 cup vodka
1/2 cup red rose petals
15 drops rose oil (or may use rosewood or geranium)

Combine the water, vodka and petals in a covered jar. Place in the sun for a day. Strain and add oil. Bottle. Recipe makes about 2 cups. Should be used within 2 weeks.

Lavender Water

Follow Rosewater Recipe, substituting 1/2 cup lavender flowers instead of roses and using 15 drops of lavender oil instead of rose oil.

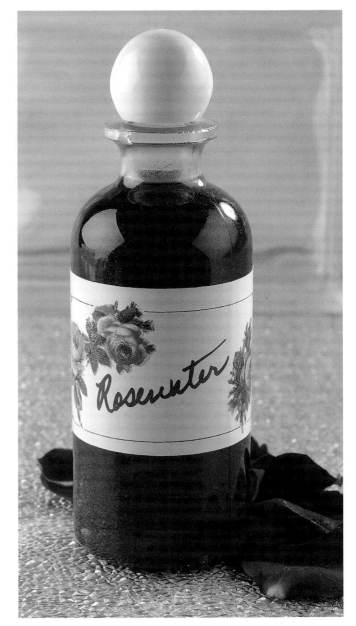

Face Oils

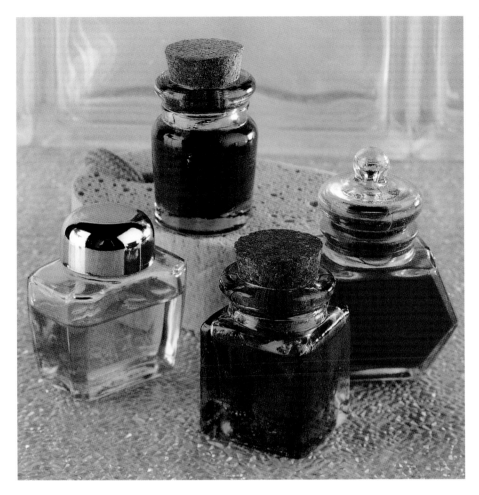

Use the following recipes after you have washed your face thoroughly. The oil acts as a moisturizer so leave the face slightly damp so the moisturizer can "lock in" the moisture and help prevent dehydration. Don't forget the neck when using moisturizer. Oftentimes, the neck can show aging faster than the face so keeping it soft and pliant is important.

RECIPE

Face Oil for Dry/Mature Skin

5 drops lavender essential oil
2 drops rosemary essential oil
2 drops sandalwood essential oil
1 oz. jojoba oil

Blend together and use as a moisturizer or night treatment.

RECIPE

Nourishing Face Oil

5 drops lavender essential oil
3 drops rosewood essential oil
2 drops patchouli essential oil
3 drops lemon essential oil
2 oz. apricot kernel oil
1 tablespoon wheat germ oil

Blend together and use as a moisturizer or night treatment. Suitable for most skin types.

Face Cream

Creams are another way to pamper your skin, moisturizing and protecting against the harsh effects of the environment.

Use the following recipe to prevent moisture loss and keep the skin smooth and pliable.

Use a massaging stroke to apply the cream to your face. This cream is especially good for all skin types.

RECIPE

Rose Moisturizing Cream

8 drops rose absolute, rosewood, or geranium essential oil
1-1/2 tablespoon beeswax
2 oz. sweet almond oil
1 oz. distilled water or rosewater
Optional Color: use 2 drops of red food coloring to tint pink.

Place the beeswax and sweet almond oil into pan or heat-resistant bowl. Place the pan or bowl into a larger pan of boiling water and stir until the mixture melts. Remove pan/bowl and slowly add distilled water or rosewater, stirring constantly. Keep stirring until mixture begins to cool. Add essential oil and stir until slightly thickened. Pour into sterilized jars.

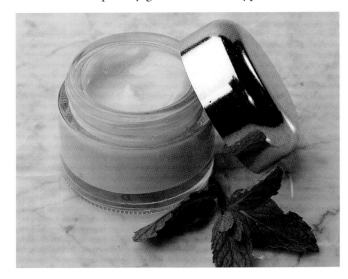

Hand Cream

We often neglect one of the most visible parts of our body, our hands. They are one of the first parts of our body to show age as well as neglect. Applying moisturizer daily - after washing hands and before going to bed - will greatly improve the appearance of your hands. Others will notice how smooth and soft they are.

The following cream recipe is especially effective as an overnight treatment. Cover dry hands with the cream and wear cotton gloves to bed so the cream is allowed to penetrate. TO APPLY: When applying the cream to your hands, use the time to massage each hand. The elbows benefit from this cream as well. Massage into each elbow with a generous amount.

RECIPE

Hand Nourishment Cream

5 drops geranium essential oil
5 drops lemon essential oil
1/2 oz. beeswax
1/2 oz. cocoa butter
5 drops evening primrose oil
2 tablespoons jojoba or sweet almond oil

1. Place the beeswax, cocoa butter, and jojoba or sweet almond oil into a heat resistant bowl. Stir over a pan of boiling water until the mixture melts.
2. Remove the bowl from the pan and when slightly cooled, add the evening primrose and essential oils, stirring constantly.
3. Stir until the mixture has thickened, then transfer to sterilized jars. Allow to cool before capping.

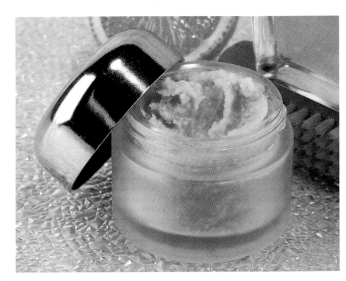

Body Moisturizing Cream

A wonderful time to moisturize the entire body is after a bath or shower. Towel dry briskly to stimulate the circulation. Then apply "Body Sherbert" over the body. It glides on, nourishing and softening the body. The fragrant scent will relax and calm you. Use large, circular movements applying a generous amount of cream.

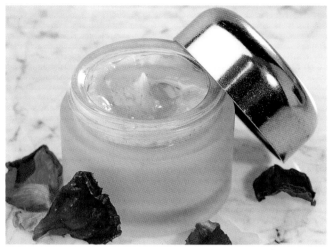

NOTE: This cream may also be used as a rich face moisturizer for nighttime. Suitable for all skin types.

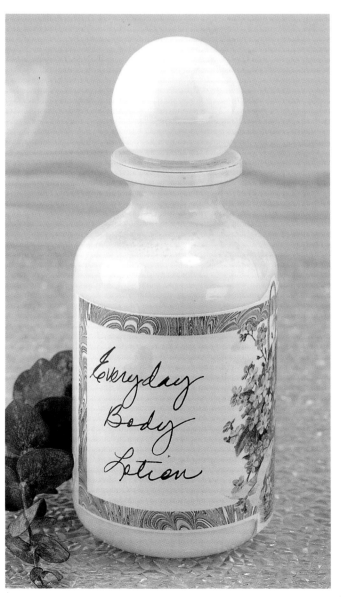

RECIPE

Rose Body Sherbert

A full body moisturizer. This recipe makes a little more than 3 oz. of cream.

8 drops of geranium or rosewood essential oil
1/2 tablespoon beeswax
2 oz. sweet almond oil
1 oz. distilled water

1. Put the beeswax and sweet almond oil into a heat resistant bowl. Stir over a pan of boiling water until the mixture melts.
2. Remove the bowl from the pan and slowly add the distilled water to the mixture, stirring constantly. Be sure to blend thoroughly so water does not separate when cooled.
3. Keep stirring while the cream begins to cool, then add the essential oils. Stir until the mixture has thickened, then transfer to sterilized jars. Allow the mixture to thoroughly cool before capping.

Everyday Body Lotion

For a fragrant day lotion, use this recipe. It's wonderful for light body fragrancing.

25 drops lavender essential oil
8 drops tea tree essential oil
10 drops rosewood
8 oz. unscented body lotion

Blend together and use all over the body for a soft feel and fragrant aroma.

Foot Care

Another neglected part of our body is our feet. To get your feet in better shape - and keep them that way - try the following. First, soak your feet in this revitalizing foot bath. It will soothe aches and itching and prepare your feet for the second recipe. If you are tired of calloused, rough skin on your feet, try the following pomade recipe. A pomade is a very thick mixture that softens and smooths.

RECIPE

Invigorating Foot Bath

1 cup distilled water
2 teaspoons unscented glycerin soap (grated)
1 teaspoon witch hazel
1/2 teaspoon tea tree essential oil

Boil water in saucepan and add soap. Stir until dissolved. Remove from heat and add witch hazel and tea tree oil, stirring until well-blended. Let cool, then bottle. This recipe makes enough for four 1/2 cup treatments. Shake well before each use. Pour into foot bath container filled with warm water. Soak feet for 15-20 minutes. Follow with moisturizing cream or, if at night before bed, with the "Overnight Foot Treatment Pomade."

RECIPE

Overnight Foot Treatment Pomade

Remedies callused, rough skin on your feet.

20 drops of rose geranium, frankincense or sandalwood
1 tablespoon beeswax
3 oz. sweet almond oil
Optional: 4 tablespoons of lanolin for very dry skin

1. Put the beeswax, sweet almond oil and lanolin, if used, into a heat resistant bowl. Stir over a pan of boiling water until melted.
2. Remove the bowl from the pan. Keep stirring while the mixture begins to cool, then add the essential oil. When thickened, transfer to sterilized jars.
3. After massaging the pomade into your feet, slip cotton socks over your feet for an ultimate make-over.

RECIPE

Perk-Me-Up Foot Oil

Try this quickie remedy for tired feet that need to keep moving!

4 drops of peppermint oil
3 oz. sweet almond oil

Blend and massage into feet. Give yourself 10 minutes to also raise your feet and relax. You'll feel like a new person!

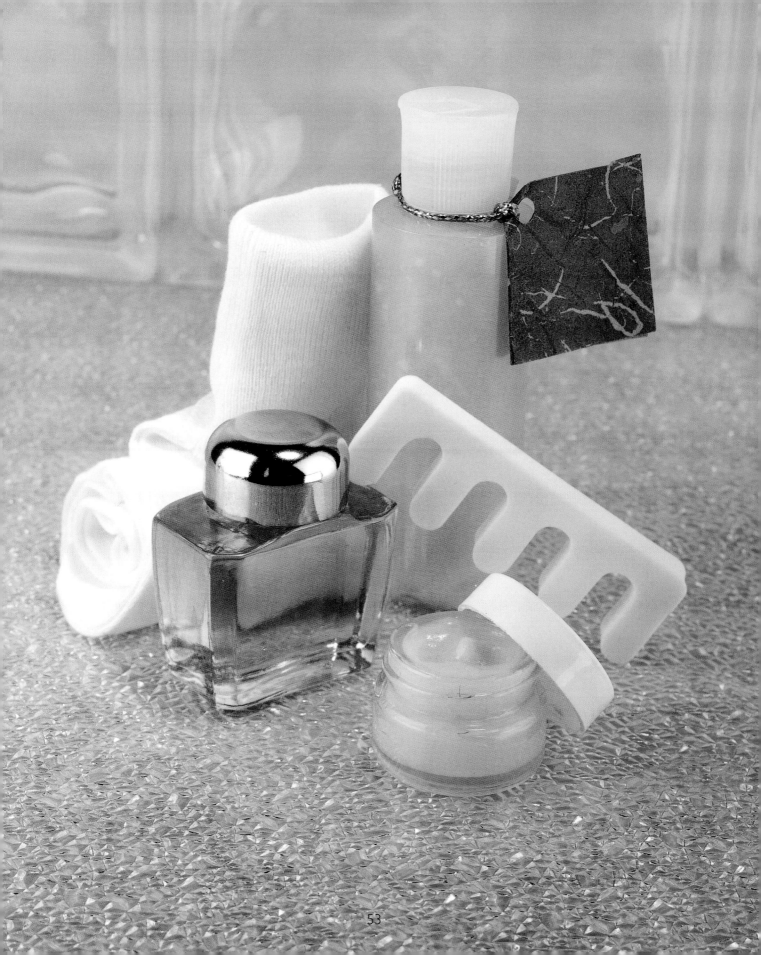

BODY
FRAGRANCING

Fragrancing your body is a personal experience. What better way to personalize your scent than by making your own perfume or cologne? It isn't hard to do and can be a very distinctive way to use aromatherapy.

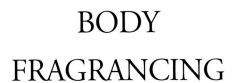

Benefits of Body Fragrancing

You can find the blend that works for you and change as your mood changes, realizing the added benefit of the essential oils on your body.

Essential oils have always been key ingredients in the world's finest perfumes. In fact, some essential oils, such as neroli or rose absolute, don't even need to be blended to create a wonderful and luxurious perfume - just put it on neat. If you're up to experimenting, however, you can create your own personal fragrance by working with various combinations of essential oils. To start you off, try some of the following blends to see what suits you best. Then experiment to your heart's content. Just remember that normally 5 drops of carrier oil should be used for every drop of essential oil.

Cologne splashes can be made by using 12 drops of essential oil to every 1 tablespoon of grain alcohol (such as Everclear or if not available, vodka).

Blend one drop at a time. You can always add more, but you can't remove an oil and may ruin a blend by hastily adding too much to cover up your mistake. Once you begin experimenting, keep track of your recipes so they can be reproduced.

REMINDER: Be sure that the oils are always diluted before applying to the skin. Even though some essential oils can be used directly on the skin (lavender, rose absolute, neroli), always do the patch test (see "Cautions" section) to make sure your skin is not adversely affected by any oil you have selected.

NOTE: Jojoba Oil is a good choice for the carrier oil mentioned in the recipes that follow. It doesn't go rancid as quickly as some of the other oils, is kind to the skin, applies easily, and tends to last longer.

RECIPES

Solid Perfume

This type of perfume is a nice alternative to regular perfume and makes an unusual gift.

1/2 cup sweet almond oil
1-1/2 teaspoons beeswax
10-15 drops essential oil (rosewood, geranium, patchouli, ylang ylang, jasmine, lavender, for example)
Optional: Vitamin E capsule

Put the sweet almond oil in heat resistant bowl and place in water bath. Melt beeswax in the oil. Add the oil from the vitamin E capsule, if desired. Mix well. Remove from heat and add essential oils. Pour into small jars and allow hardening before capping.

RECIPES

Garden Delight Perfume

3 drops rose absolute
6 drops lavender
5 drops patchouli
1/2 oz. jojoba oil

Combine and bottle in sterilized glass container.

RECIPES

Refreshing After-Bath Splash

(Use this splash also as a light cologne.)

1/2 cup distilled water
1/4 cup vodka
15 drops lavender essential oil
4 drops sandalwood essential oil

Combine together in a glass bottle (spritzer) and shake until well mixed.

RECIPES

Cologne Splash Recipe #1

Use the "Garden Delight Perfume Recipe" – but substitute 1 oz. grain alcohol for 1/2 oz. jojoba oil. May also add 1-2 drops of cinnamon. Add essential oils to the bottle first, then add alcohol to avoid cloudiness. May be bottled in clear glass perfume bottle, preferably a spritzer since dabbing the cologne may cause the skin to sting.

Cologne Splash Recipe #2

Combine 1/4 cup vodka and 1/4 cup distilled water. Add 1 teaspoon jojoba oil and 10 drops of any essential oil. Place all ingredients into a spray bottle and shake until well-mixed.

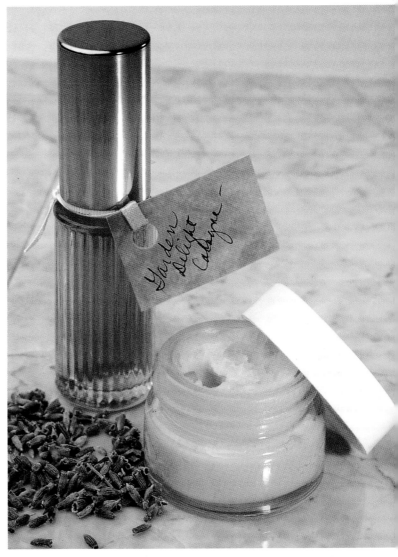

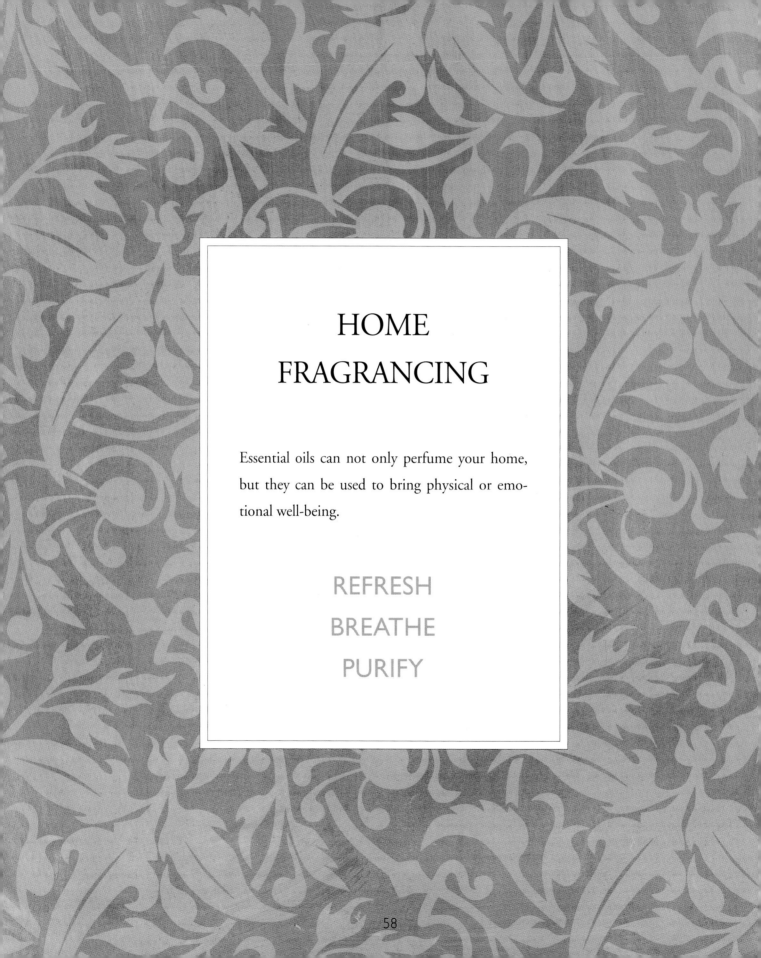

HOME
FRAGRANCING

Essential oils can not only perfume your home, but they can be used to bring physical or emotional well-being.

REFRESH

BREATHE

PURIFY

Ways to Perfume Your Home

Perfuming your home with essential oils can be managed through a number of ways.

Aromatic diffusers: These contain a little glass nebulizer attached to an air pump and work without heat. A fine mist is released into the room. These can be expensive to buy and some caution must be used since the oils can land on furniture and damage them.

Commercial burners: These are also known as simmer pots. They normally consist of a small container that should be filled with water and essential oil added. The container is then placed above a candle or light. When the flame burns (or the light becomes warm), the oil is heated and disperses its scent throughout the room.

Other diffusers: These can be as simple as a brass or ceramic ring that is filled with essential oil and fits on top of a light bulb; or a plug-in that has pads to hold the essential oil. All do a nice job of diffusing the scent of the essential oils into the room.

Room Spray: Another way to refresh the rooms in your home (or car) is to use a spray bottle that has a combination of distilled water and essential oils. Whatever the mood you desire, whatever therapy is needed, this method works with very little effort or cost. Try the following recipes. Use any size spray bottle, from 4 oz. to 16 oz.

CAUTION: Just remember to use caution with any equipment that heats up. Pure essential oils are flammable and must be attended while they are burning. Always ensure that the burners, diffusers, and any equipment using essential oils are out of the reach of children and pets.

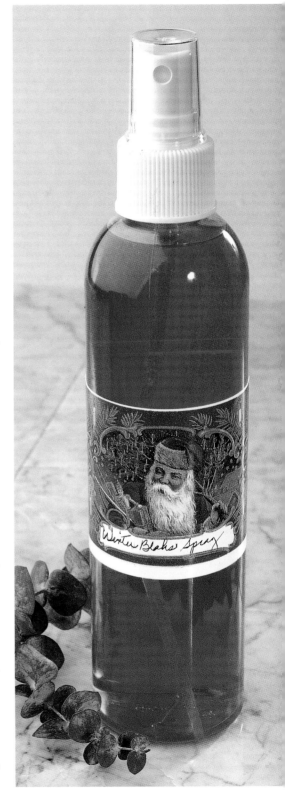

❧ ROOM SPRAY BASIC RECIPE

20-25 drops of essential oil
16 oz. distilled water

Add the oil to the water in a sterilized spray bottle. Shake well before any spraying is done into the air. Avoid spraying directly on wooden furniture. You may spray bed sheets, pillows, handkerchiefs and tissues with this spray so that you can inhale the scent at any time.

❧ ROOM SPRAY BLENDS

Any of the oils listed below may be used alone with distilled water in the spray bottle. If you would prefer to just use a 4 oz. bottle, add 5-6 drops of the chosen oil to the distilled water.

Sick Room Disinfecting Spray: Tea tree, juniper, rosemary, eucalyptus, lemon, or combination.

Floral Spray: Lavender, geranium, patchouli, rose absolute, rosewood, or combination.

Invigorating Spray: Peppermint, lemon, rosemary, or combination.

Calming Spray: Frankincense, chamomile, sandalwood, lavender, or combination.

Winter Blahs Spray: Sweet orange, lavender, lemon, ylang ylang, rose absolute, clary sage, frankincense, or a combination of 3-4 oils.

RECIPES

Colds/Flu Decongesting Spray

7 drops eucalyptus
7 drops frankincense
7 drops tea tree
4 drops rosemary

Add to 16 oz. distilled water in spritzer. Shake well before each use.

Citrus Fresh Spray

(Great for Kitchens)

5 drops bergamot
8 drops grapefruit
8 drops lemon

Add to 16 oz. distilled water in spritzer. Shake well before each use.

Romance is in the Air Spray

(A sensual spray for the bedroom)

10 drops jasmine
5 drops patchouli
5 drops sandalwood
5 drops ylang ylang

Add to 16 oz. distilled water in spritzer. Shake well before each use.

Long Distance Driving Spray

(This recipe is for a smaller container so you can keep it in your car.)

2 drops rosemary
2 drops sweet orange
1 drop eucalyptus
1 drop lemon

Add to 4 oz. distilled water in spray bottle. Shake well before each use.

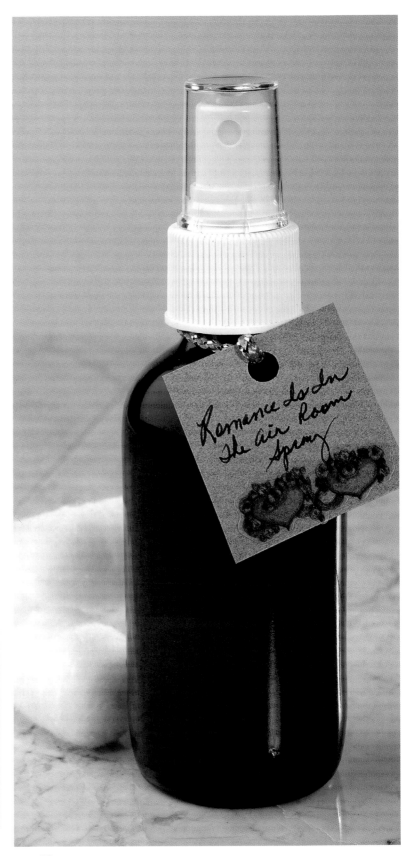

Candles as Mood Enhancers

Another wonderful way to enjoy the inhalation of essential oils and at the same time scent your home is to use candles. Buy unscented pillar candles in the color and size desired. Light the wick and allow some of the wax to melt. Blow out the flame then add several drops of essential oil in the melted wax before lighting the candle again. As the wax is warmed, the scent of the essential oil will be released. Three to four drops of essential oil should last 1-2 hours.

There are many wonderful aromatherapy candles on the market today. They are available in single scents and mood blends. You can make your own by using paraffin or beeswax in molds or containers and scenting the wax before it hardens.

Whichever way you choose to go, candles add a great deal. Use them in all rooms. Bathe by candlelight using the same or complementary oils in the bath water as well as in the candle. Aromatherapy is all about enjoying the essence of the moment - candles definitely enhance the mood with their flickering light and the lovely aroma of essential oils.

❧ BLENDS TO USE WITH CANDLES

Blend together in a bottle and add 3-4 drops every 1-2 hours for lasting aroma.

Energizer: 4 drops rosemary, 2 drops peppermint, 1 drop lemon

Holiday Joy: 3 drops frankincense, 7 drops sweet orange, 5 drops juniper

Meditative State: 2 drops frankincense, 2 drops sandalwood, 5 drops tangerine

Happy Moods: 5 drops orange, 2 drops peppermint, 4 drops sandalwood or 2 drops rosemary, 5 drops bergamot, 3 drops lavender

Sensual Evening: 4 drops sandalwood, 6 drops ylang ylang, 5 drops sweet orange

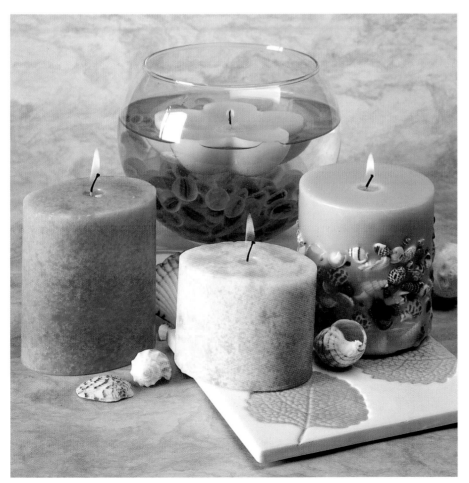

AROMATHERAPY
ON-THE-GO

Many times small illnesses when you're away from home can spoil the whole experience. You carry medications when you're going on a trip to take care of headaches, minor aches and pains, stomachaches, etc. Why not make up a kit of aromatherapy remedies as a first aid kit for travel-related problems? These travel kits may just make the difference between a good trip and one spoiled by nagging problems.

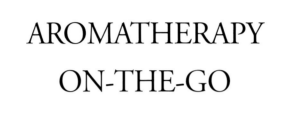

UPLIFTING

CALM

SOOTHE

Travel by Plane

Many problems can occur when traveling by plane, both during the time you are flying and upon arrival, especially if you are traveling across time zones and in the airplane for more than 2-3 hours. Disorientation, swollen ankles, dehydration, loss of appetite, and confusion caused by a change of time zone are all symptoms of jet lag. Another interrupter can be travel sickness, a nausea caused either by motion or fear of the journey itself.

Try these recipes to take on your next trip. You may inhale the oils from the bottle, a hankie or tissue, or use in a diffuser you take along. Use them in a bath or massage to get the multiple benefits that either afford.

CAUTION: Be sure you have any oils in tightly capped, dark bottles. There are boxes available from some aromatherapists, but if you tighten the lids securely on the bottles and then place in a sealable plastic bag, the oils should remain intact. Try to keep them upright in your suitcase and carry them on board with you - to decrease likelihood of them being broken - but also to use while on the plane.

RECIPE

Jet Lag Remedy

Two effects are needed when experiencing jet lag: calming effects to assist the body in relaxing enough to sleep and uplifting effects to assist the body in feeling alert and energized.

Calming: Add up to 8 drops of clary sage, geranium, lavender, or rose essential oils to 1 tablespoon of carrier oil.
• A firm, energetic foot massage with the above oils will boost energy. These oils may also be added to the bath.

Uplifting: Add up to 8 drops of orange, peppermint, rosemary, lemon, or eucalyptus essential oils to 1 tablespoon of carrier oil.

• For sleep, use a gentle shoulder. Massage or foot massage with oil. Also may be added to the bath.

• As an Inhalant: May also use 2 drops of any of preceding oils on a hankie, tissue or cotton ball and inhale.

RECIPE

Travel Sickness Remedy

Place 2 drops of any of the following oils on a hankie, tissue or cotton ball and inhale. Use lavender, lemon, sweet orange, or peppermint.

These fresh-smelling oils will help calm the stomach and mind.
DO NOT USE MASSAGE TECHNIQUES WITH THIS REMEDY.

HINT: Hankies, tissues, or cotton balls can be moistened with essential oils prior to taking a trip and stored in airtight plastic bags. Then all you need to do is just open the bag and inhale. Be sure you label each bag as to its contents.

Travel by Car

Traveling by car can be a pleasure or a pure test of will power. Essential oils can help ease the difficulties often experienced with road travel. Try these ideas out on your next trip.

• Use spritzer bottles to which you have added distilled water and a few drops of peppermint, rosemary, or lemon (4-5 drops of essential oil to 4 oz. of distilled water) to aid the tired driver. The blend can be sprayed into the air or on a tissue and then can be inhaled to aid alertness.

• You may also wish to moisten a hankie, tissue, or cotton ball with a couple of drops of essential oils and just inhale as needed. Good oils to use in this way include lavender, to keep cool and calm in traffic jams; basil to help you stay alert when you're sleepy or tired; or peppermint to soothe an upset stomach.

• Use the travel sickness recipe in the section above to aid people who experience car sickness.

❦ FIRST AID KIT

Whether traveling by plane or car or other modes of transportation, a first aid kit will always come in handy. To make one, include: 1/8 oz. dark-colored vials containing your essential oils, a bottle of carrier base oil, empty spray bottle, small bottle of distilled water, Lavender First Aid Ointment (recipe, page 71), handkerchief, and a nice fabric pouch to hold all of this. You could also make a booklet that lists ailments and their remedies. Keeping one in the home is also a good idea. The following treatments are designed for minor ailments and should never replace medical attention.

A first aid kit can include remedies for the following:
Minor cuts, abrasions and sores
Minor burns
Insect bites and stings
Headaches
Muscular aches and pains
Sore throat
Congestion
Colds and coughs
Sleeplessness
Jet Lag
Travel sickness

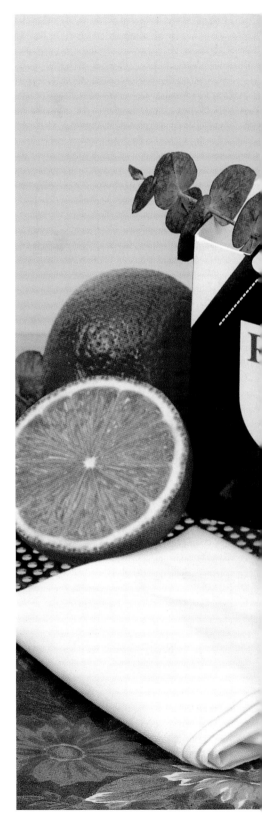

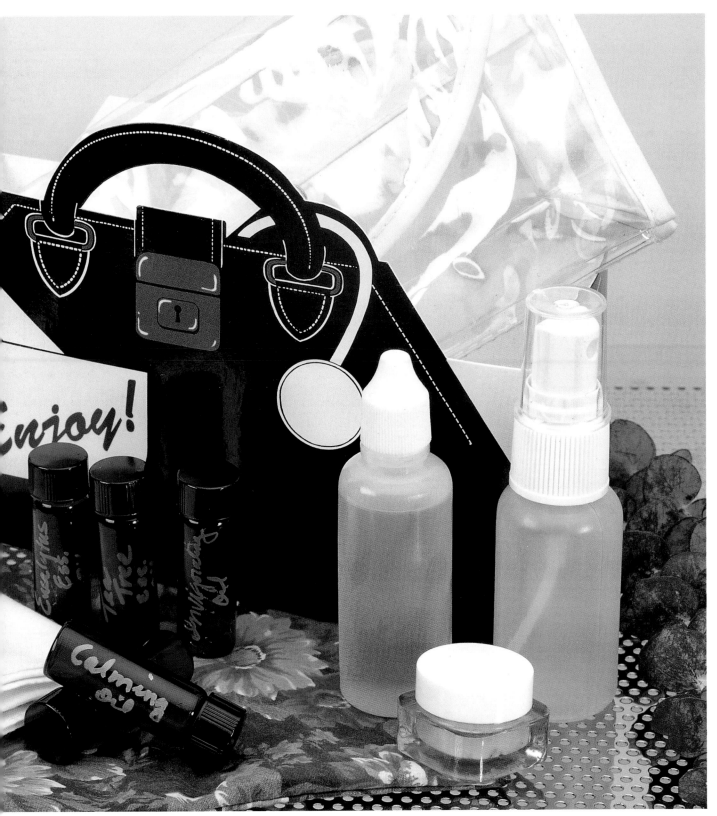

Aromatherapy First Aid Kit
Instruction Booklet

Make this great little booklet to slip into your Travel First Aid Kit. If you wish, you can photocopy the pages given here, cut them out, and assemble into a booklet.

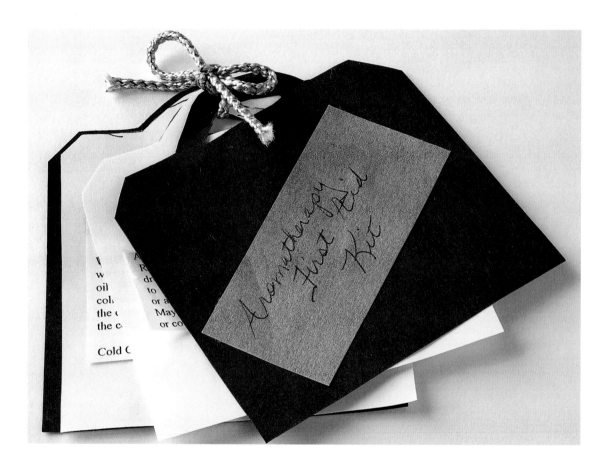

Supplies needed:
1 piece of black card stock - 4" x 8"
1 piece of gold card stock - 3" x 1-1/2"
1 piece of 12" gold braid ribbon
Craft knife
Black fine tip permanent marker
Copied pages from this chapter of Ailments and Remedies

How To:
1. Trace pattern for medicine bag on to black card stock to make 1 front piece and 1 back piece.
2. Cut out the pattern and then use a craft knife to cut out space between the handle and the bag.
3. Use the black marker to write "Aromatherapy First Aid Kit" on the piece of gold card stock . Glue the gold piece at a slant on the front of one of the black medicine bag pieces.
4. Cut out the 12 pages with Ailment/Rx for the booklet. Use a craft knife to cut out the handle for each page.
5. Assemble ailment/remedy sheets between covers and tie together with gold braid ribbon.

Remedies

Ailment: Jet Lag

Rx:
To assist the body in relaxing enough to sleep, add up to 8 drops of clary sage, geranium, lavender, or rose essential oils to 1 tablespoon of carrier oil. Massage into shoulder or feet or add to the bath.
May also use 2 drops of any of the above oils on a hankie, tissue, or cotton ball and inhale.

Ailment: Travel Sickness

Rx:
Place 2 drops of any of the following oils on a hankie, tissue or cotton ball and inhale. Use lavender, lemon, sweet orange, or peppermint.
These fresh-smelling oils will help calm the stomach and mind.
DO NOT USE MASSAGE TECHNIQUES WITH THIS REMEDY.

Ailment: Minor Cuts, Abrasions, Sores

Rx:
Oils to Use: Bergamot, geranium, lavender, tea tree, chamomile
Application: Clean affected area with cool water then apply a cold compress made with 4 drops of essential oils.
Lavender and tea tree may be used directly on the wound without diluting.

Ailment: Minor Burns

Rx:
Oils to Use: Geranium, chamomile, lavender, tea tree
Application: Immerse affected area in cold water then apply lavender oil directly on the burn. A cold compress may be made with 4 drops of lavender oil and 2 drops of chamomile.
Lavender and tea tree may be used directly on the burn.

Remedies

Ailment: Insect Bites and Stings

Rx:
Oils to Use: Lavender or tea tree
Application: Dab a drop of lavender or tea tree on the affected area. If swollen, apply a cold compress made with 2 drops each of lavender and chamomile oils.

Ailment: Headaches

Rx:
Oils to Use: geranium, lavender, peppermint, rosemary
Application: Blend up to 8 drops of geranium, lavender, peppermint or rosemary, or a blend of the oils, in 1 tablespoon of carrier oil. Massage with circular motions on the temples, forehead and the base of the skull. NOTE: If the headache is caught in the initial stage of pain, just uncapping and smelling the essential oil will sometimes stop the headache from developing.
This blend may also be used in a bath.

Ailment: Muscular Aches and Pains

Rx:
Oils to Use: eucalyptus, juniper, lavender, rosemary
Application: Add up to 8 drops of eucalyptus, juniper, lavender, or rosemary, or a blend of the oils, to 1 tablespoon of carrier oil. Use in bath and/or gently massage the achy area.

Ailment: Sore Throat

Rx:
Oils to Use: clary sage, lavender, peppermint, sandalwood, tea tree
Application: Blend 8 drops of clary sage, lavender, peppermint, sandalwood, or tea tree, or a blend of the oils, in a 1 tablespoon of carrier oil. Gently stroke down the neck then use large, gentle circular movements on either side of the neck.
This blend may also be added to the bath.
A warm compress using 4 drops of essential oil may be applied to the neck.

Ailment: Congestion
Rx:
Oils to Use: rosemary, eucalyptus, frankincense, peppermint
Application: Blend 2 drops each of rosemary and eucalyptus and 1 drop frankincense with 1 table-spoon sweet almond oil. Place the blend on the hands and gently stroke down the nose, out to the ears, and down the neck. It may also help to use deep, circular pressures at the base of the skull, fol-lowed by squeezing the eyebrows, and putting pres-sure on the eyebrows, forehead, and base of the nose.

You may also use 2 drops of eucalyptus, peppermint, or rosemary on a hankie/tissue and inhale. For night-time relief, keep the hankie/tissue by your pillow so you can breathe in the vapors of the essential oil as you sleep.

Ailment: Colds and Coughs
Rx:
Oils to Use: bergamot, eucalyptus, frankincense, lavender, peppermint, rosemary, sandalwood, tea tree
Application: Blend up to 8 drops of bergamot, eucalyptus, frankincense, lavender, peppermint, rosemary, sandalwood, or tea tree (or a combination – for example, 4 drops bergamot with 2 drops each of tea tree and eucalyptus) with 1 tablespoon of car-rier oil. Stroke the chest with the blend then gently massage neck and face.
Use up to 5 drops of any of the above essential oils to bath water. May also use the blend above.
To 8 oz. of distilled water in a spritzer bottle, add 5 drops of any of the above essential oils and use as air freshener. May also be used to spritz pillow.

Use this for your own notes

Ailment: Sleeplessness

Rx:
Oils to Use: lavender, roman chamomile, neroli
Application: Blend 4 drops lavender, 2 drops each of Roman chamomile, and neroli with 1 table-spoon sweet almond oil. Use as a slow, rhythmic massage on the back with gentle stroking. May also follow with a bath using the blend.
Place 2-4 drops of lavender, neroli, or sweet orange on the pillow to encourage sleep.

HEALING
ROUTINES

There are numerous ways aromatherapy can be used for healing of the physical body.

WELL-BEING

HEALING

RELIEF

Ointments

An ointment is a type of salve that is applied to the skin for healing or for cosmetic purposes. The consistency is solid or firm to the touch. Essential oils are added to a base/carrier oil along with an ingredient that solidifies the blend.

- To make a basic ointment:

  Heat 2 tablespoons of sweet almond oil in a pan and place the pan into a larger pan of boiling water. Add 4 tablespoons of anhydrous lanolin to the sweet almond oil and blend. When well-blended, mix in 15-20 drops of essential oil and allow the mixture to cool. Pour into containers.

Ointments are good to use as overnight treatments or as salves to put on injured or achy areas.

RECIPE

Lavender First Aid Ointment

Try this ointment recipe as an addition to your medicine chest, first aid kit, or travel kit. It makes a welcome gift as well.

4 tablespoons base/carrier oil, such as
sweet almond or jojoba
3 tablespoons beeswax
3 teaspoons cocoa butter
2 teaspoons anhydrous lanolin
Vitamin E capsule (puncture to release oil)
20 drops lavender essential oil
15 drops sandalwood essential oil

Combine sweet almond oil, beeswax, cocoa butter and lanolin and heat thoroughly in the top of a double boiler. Remove from heat. Add the vitamin E (puncturing the capsule to release the oil), lavender and sandalwood oils, and beat well. Pour into jars and allow mixture to cool before capping.

This recipe keeps well and should last up to a year. The ointment is very effective for burns, chapped lips, and cold sores. I have a friend who has made this recipe exclusively for her brother-in-law who had suffered a great deal from cold sores. He could find nothing to really help - until he tried this ointment. If he uses it at the first sign of the cold sore, he has no pain and the sore heals quickly. It's a must- have to keep with you and to stock in your medicine chest!

Compresses

Compresses are an age-old remedy and are very effective in using essential oils to relieve pain and reduce inflammation. A warm compress can be made by filling a bowl with hot water and adding up to 6 drops of essential oil. Stir, then place a face cloth on the water's surface to collect a film of oil. Wring out the excess water and apply the cloth to the affected area until it has cooled. Repeat until the compress has been used for 10-20 minutes. Use warm compresses to ease backache, abdominal pains, rheumatism and arthritis, sore throat or congestion due to colds and flu.

Cold compresses are made in a similar way, using very cold water rather than hot water. This type of compress is useful for headaches (apply to forehead or back of neck), cramps, sprains, strains, and other swollen conditions.

❧ HERBAL COMPRESS

You can make an herbal compress using flax seed and lavender essential oil that smells heavenly and helps with headaches. Follow these instructions:

Supplies needed for one herbal compress:

8-1/2" x 10" piece of interfacing (or some other "breathable" material)*

10-1/8" x 10-3/4" piece of fabric

1/2 cup of flax seed

1 tablespoon of fixative (like Baby Magic™** or oak moss)

10 drops lavender essential oil

Instructions:

1. Put fixative in mortar and pestle or bowl. Moisten with essential oil and blend thoroughly.
2. Add mixture to flax seed. Set aside.
3. Sew 3 sides of the interfacing together and fill with scented flax seed. Stitch 4th side closed.
4. Sew 3 sides of fabric together, right sides facing. Turn right side out.
5. Put scented bag into fabric cover.
6. Turn raw edge of unsewed end over twice (so no raw selvage shows) and stitch with machine.

*I used interfacing as the inner bag because the scented flax seed can easily be smelled, and you can refresh the bag by spraying it with distilled water to which you've added lavender oil without staining the fabric. Feel free to experiment with fabrics of your choice.

**Baby Magic (TM) is a commercial fixative that I purchase from Lavender Lane in Sacramento, California. I like it because it is not messy, but you may use orris root, oakmoss, or any other fixative you normally use with potpourri. Or you may just scent the flax seed itself and add lavender flowers to get a gentle fragrance.

Inhalations and Facial Steams

Inhalations are invaluable for easing respiratory problems, sore throats, and coughs. Fill a large bowl with boiling water and add 2-6 drops of essential oil. Lean over the bowl, and cover your head with a towel to trap the steam for 5-10 minutes. Take deep breaths. Remember to shut your eyes since the vapor from the oils can sting them. For respiratory problems, use up to three times a day. Discontinue if you feel any discomfort. This method directly affects the respiratory system and the blood supply. CAUTION: If you have asthma or broken capillaries, the inhalation method should not be used.

This method is also an effective way to open the pores on your face in order to deep clean the skin. Do not use more than once a week.

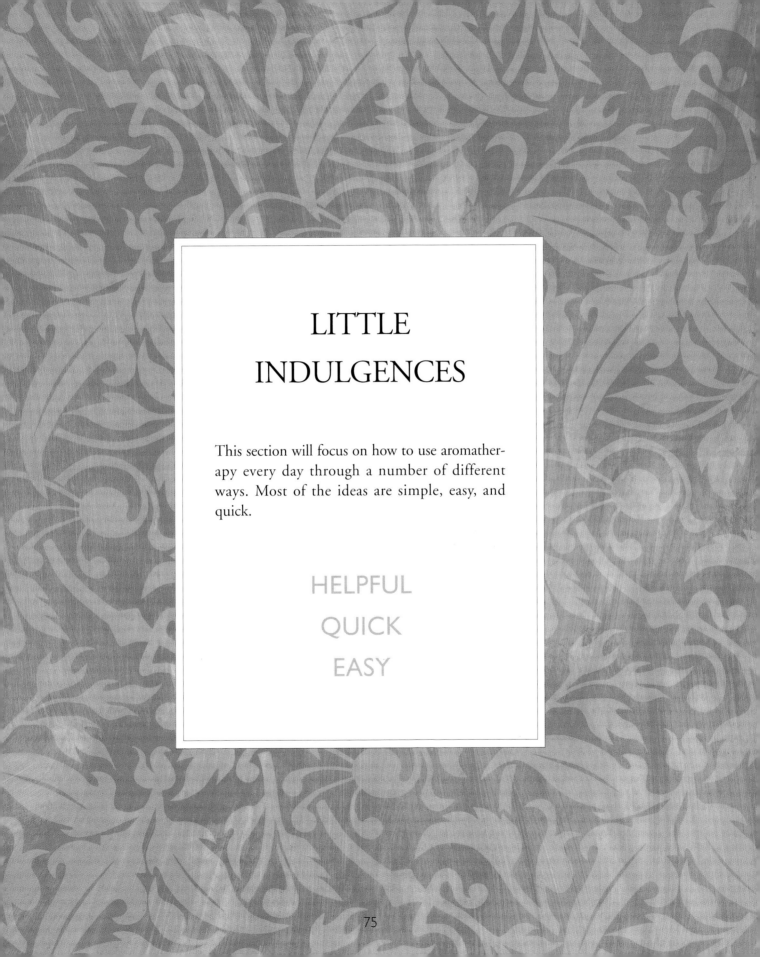

LITTLE
INDULGENCES

This section will focus on how to use aromatherapy every day through a number of different ways. Most of the ideas are simple, easy, and quick.

HELPFUL

QUICK

EASY

Scented Shells

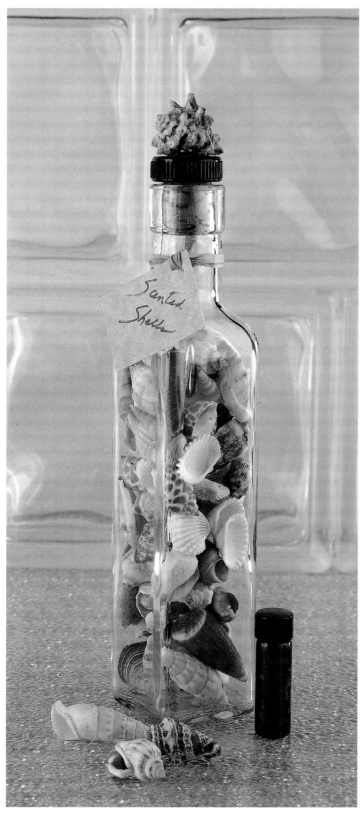

Even though this idea is simple, the scented shells are both pretty and fragrant. Use all types of shells that you have bought or collected yourself. Even pebbles from the beach and rivers add a nice texture.

Any essential oil may be used - the fresh, light fragrances usually work best. Just put a few drops of the oil on each shell/pebble. Place in a closed container and let the shells/pebbles "marinate" for a few days. Then place in a lovely container, such as a bag, box, or bottle. If used as a gift, attach a spare bottle of the essential oil so the recipient can freshen the shells.

This makes a lovely gift for people who are water-oriented.

Scented Pine Cones

Another gift idea - and a special treat for yourself as well - is to scent pine cones for use both as fire starters and as a fragrant throw-on for the fire. Just put a few drops of a favorite holiday scent - or blend a special one - on each pine cone. Place in a closed container for a few days then display in a basket ready to go by the hearth. It's always a good idea if using the scented pine cones for a gift to include a spare bottle of essential oil for refreshing.

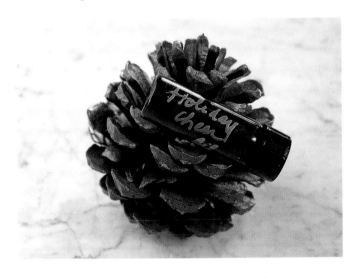

RECIPE

Holiday Cheer Refresher Oil

30 drops sweet orange
15 drops rosewood
15 drops frankincense
10 drops juniper
5 drops eucalyptus

Place oils in 1/8 oz. dark, glass bottle. Cap tightly and label.

*This recipe may also be used to scent candles.

Moth Sachets

When combining dried herbs known for their insect-repelling nature (such as pennyroyal, bay, rosemary, wormwood, lavender, etc.), add a few drops of the insect-repelling essential oils - cedarwood, lavender, lemon, clove). Package in sealable tea bags, muslin, squares of cloth. Makes a very nice accessory gift to go along with a clothing item, blankets, or other items that are likely to be stored over the summer months.

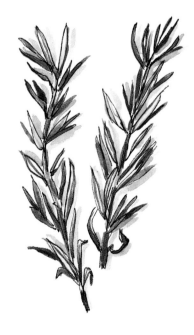

Carpet Freshener

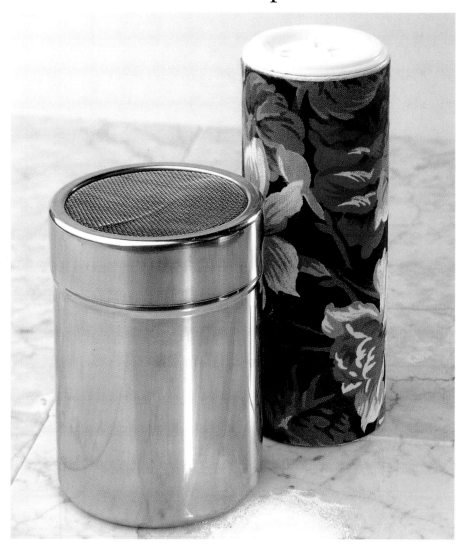

To freshen carpets, use 25 drops of essential oil such as lavender, cinnamon, rosewood, or sweet orange to 2 cups of borax. Blend well making sure all oil is crushed well and evenly distributed. Place in shaker can and apply to carpet or rug.

Essential Oils Everywhere...

Add drops of your favorite essential oil to: trash compactor or garbage can; stale potpourri; cardboard tube of toilet paper; stationery; hair brush or comb right before using; final rinse cycle in your washer then on cloth for dryer; dishwashing water (lemon is great!); soap for washing floors (20 drops per 2 gallons of water); humidifier water (1-9 drops).

Car Fresheners

Put a few drops of lavender, eucalyptus, or peppermint oil on cotton balls or tissues and place in the rear window or the dashboard of your car. The aroma will freshen the air, cool and soothe and relax the occupants.

Plane Remedy

When ankles swell during your plane trip or upon arrival at your destination, apply a compress of lavender to your feet. Keep a hankie with 5 drops of lavender on it in a plastic bag. Use it as your compress. Then massage both the front and back of the leg in an upward direction toward the calf.

Leg Calmer

For nervous, twitchy legs, put 15 drops of chamomile essential oil in 2 tablespoons of base/carrier oil. Massage legs and feet with the oil. Works well on adults and children alike.

Toilet Seat Sanitizer

Sanitize toilet seats with a tissue to which you've added a few drops of lavender and eucalyptus. Works on basins and tubs as well. Great travel companion.

Sunburn Reliever

Take a cool shower or bath then apply lavender oil neat over the affected areas.

Hair Care

You can add essential oil to your shampoo or conditioner. For a hair rinse, use a scented vinegar and rinse thoroughly. The rinse helps remove all residue from the hair and makes it smell nice at the same time.

Massage a few drops of rosemary essential oil into your hair before shampooing. It will act as a growth tonic, will condition and add body to the hair. If you use a drop or two of the oil on your hairbrush, it will prevent static electricity.

PACKAGING
IDEAS

After you've finished your special blends, you'll want to share them with others. To give one of your creations as a gift will be a special treat for the recipient. People love to receive unusual gifts that turn out to be treasures. Creatively packaging your gifts will set the right tone for their special-ness. Make them look appealing and fabulous by following some of the ideas that follow. The ideas will spark your own creativity for endless ways to dazzle others with your gifts.

TREASURES

SPECIAL

PRETTY

Containers

❧ BOTTLES

Bottles will be the right choice for many of the ideas in this book. You may choose previously used bottles as long as they have been sterilized by a hot washing by hand or in the dishwasher. Look for unusual ones at garage sales, antique stores, auctions. Many mail order companies and import stores have a wide and exciting collection of bottles.

• Massage oils, bath oils, remedy blends, perfumes can all be put in exotic, colored, or clear bottles, new or old, as long as they are stored in dark, cool areas.

• Travel kit blends can be placed in dark, glass bottles or for short term use, plastic bottles (never store your essential oils – unless mixed with a carrier oil – in plastic containers).

• Room fresheners can be placed in plastic bottles with spray attachments.

❧ JARS

Jars in assorted sizes are ideal for creams. Bath salts can be displayed in jars or bottles, tins, plastic bags, even envelopes you can make yourself.

❧ BOXES & BASKETS

Fancy boxes or baskets are always a good choice for packaging your creations. Even ordinary cardboard boxes can become eye-catchers just by spray painting then covering with wallpaper or self-sticking fabric, decoupaging, rubber stamping, or stenciling.

If using a box or basket for a gift collection, try using scented tissue paper as a liner. Use the blend or single fragrance of your gift. Since essential oils and carrier oils can stain paper, try using several drops in a grain alcohol base in a spray bottle to scent the paper. Spray lightly, allow to dry, and the alcohol will evaporate without leaving a mark. This can also be sprayed on gift wrap, ribbons or bows.

You may also apply several drops of the essential oil that is your dominant scent to the inside of the box. The cardboard will absorb the oil and the scent will last for a long time.

❧ ACCENTS

You can accent the bottles with ribbons, raffia, dried or silk flowers – the choices are endless. Be sure to label each bottle with the description and use of the contents. Seal bottles with sealing wax for an extra special touch.

Gift Collections

When combining several products together, choose a theme for the gift collection. The container that will hold the collection should fit the theme and enhance it. This can be a basket, a dish, a bag that can be used as an accessory for your products or is a gift in itself.

Fill the container with filler that will hold the products in place and complement the container. Examples of filler include excelsior, shredded paper, confetti, or tissue paper. You can also use fabric as a liner. If the container is deep, use crumpled newspaper or packing peanuts as a base and put the filler on top to conceal it. Dried or silk flowers/leaves can be used as accents for the scent, color, or theme of the gift.

Use netting, tulle, cellophane or heavy plastic wrap as a final wrapping to keep everything in place.

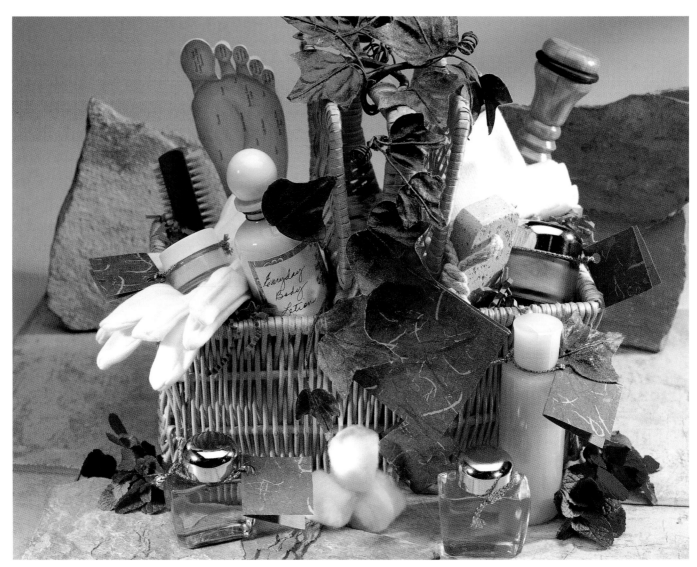

Sealing Bottles

Bottled bath oils, massage oils, scented vinegars, and bath salts can be easily sealed with sealing wax. Sealing wax will make your bottle leak-proof and attractive. The wax contains a rubber compound that acts like plastic.

To seal bottle:

1. Place the sealing wax in an old pot or a throwaway, foil container. Place in a skillet of water to create a double boiler. Heat until wax melts.

2. Place a cork into top of bottle. Wrap a piece of cord or ribbon around neck of bottle, then bring it over top of bottle and back down. Tape in place to hold.

3. Dip bottle top into wax and then lift. Set bottle aside to cool.

4. Trim cord or ribbon if necessary, allowing at least 1" of cord or ribbon showing. To open bottle, grasp end of cord and pull to break the seal of the wax.

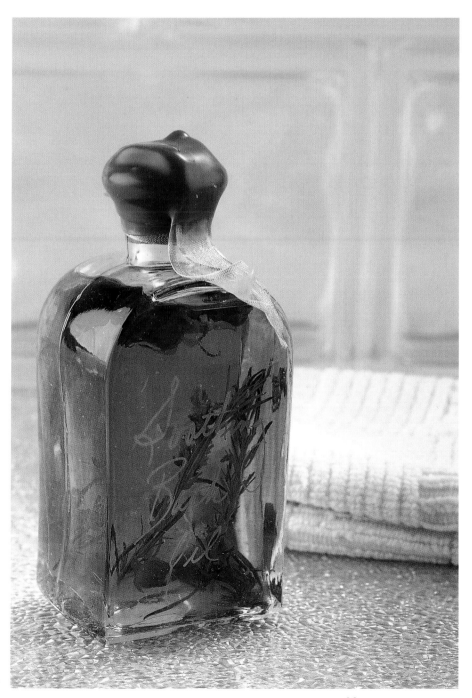

Labeling

Always label all products, whether you are keeping them for yourself or giving as gifts. Write the name of the product on the label - if using adhesive labels, waterproof them by rubbing a white candle over the writing to produce a wax coating that will be resistant to moisture. Another idea is to write with a permanent marker directly on the bottle. Use paint pens in various colors available from craft, art supply, and stationery stores. If you use a computer, there are many label programs to produce a variety of sizes and shapes. Copy on to colored paper, use card stock, or cardboard - whatever fits the gift you are giving. Another way to individualize the label is to use rubber stamping or stenciling. The possibilities are endless. Ready-made labels can also be purchased at craft shops or through mail order.

Attach a card to the product that lists ingredients and any special usage instructions. Or make up a special card that is included with the gift that lists all the products, their ingredients and usage.

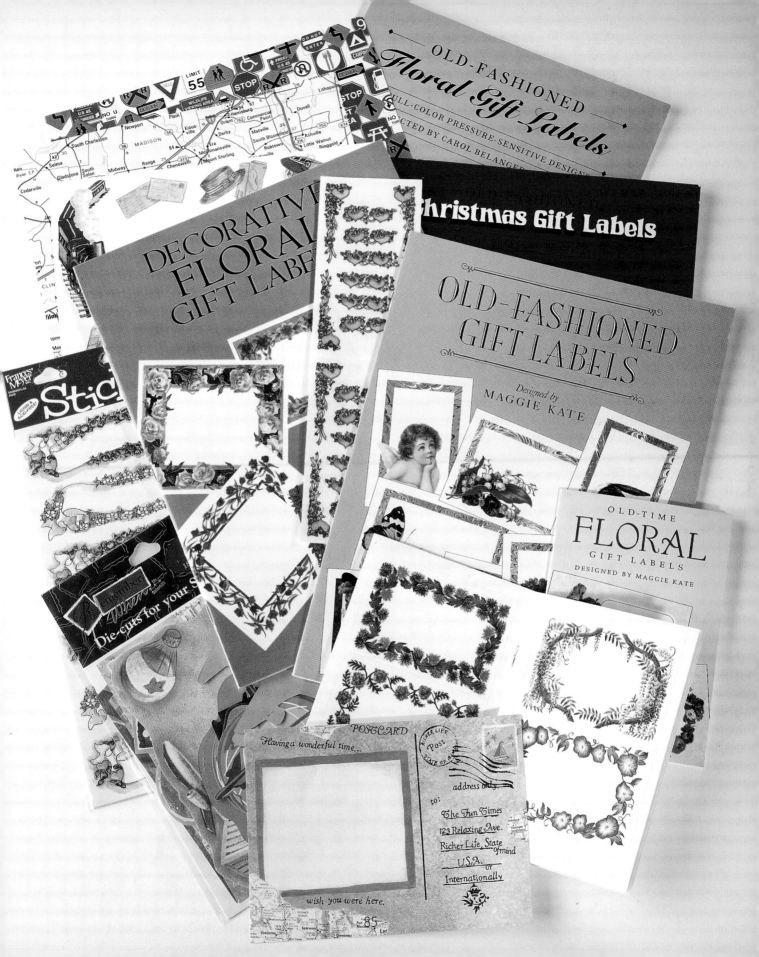

Envelopes

❧ ENVELOPE FOR BATH SALTS

Photocopy the pattern shown. Cut out and trace the pattern on a sheet of paper with the appropriate theme. (I bought 8 1/2" by 11" sheets that are in the scrapbook section of craft stores.) Cut out the pattern and fold sides in first then fold in the bottom flap. Glue bottom flap to sides. Fold top of envelope over the bottom flap. After contents are inserted, glue top flap to bottom flap and label front.

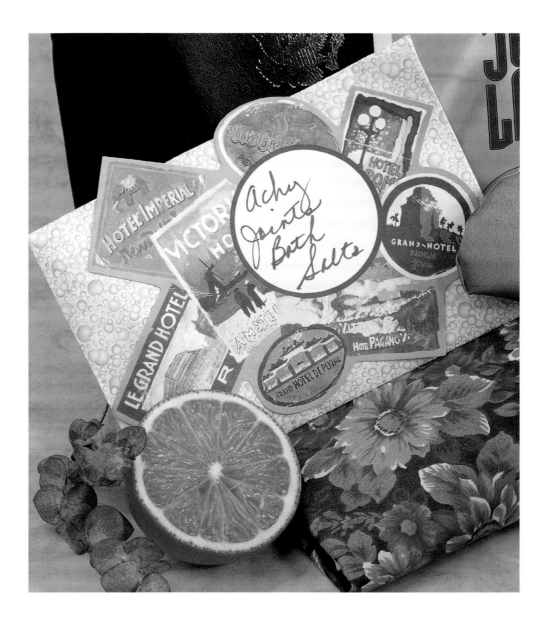

Pattern for Envelope

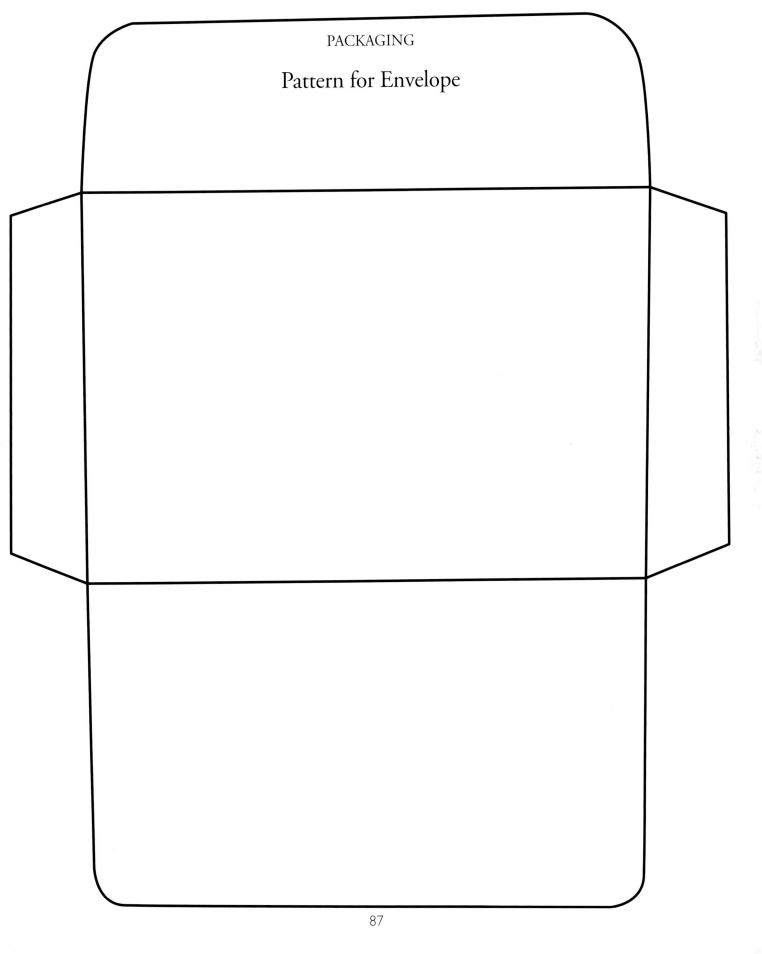

GIFT
COLLECTIONS

Does a friend or family member have a birthday or some other special event approaching? Are you tired of going from store to store to find just the right gift? The recipes in this book can be combined to make wonderful gift collections. Just pick a central theme and make up the recipes that capture that theme. Pick a container that fits the theme. Even better is to find a container that can be a gift in itself: an unusual basket, a wooden box, a jewelry case, a fabric bag. Use dried or silk flowers as filler or accents. Add a candle or accessory to use with the gift. What about a book on the topic? The following pages will help spark your own ideas in combining and individualizing gifts.

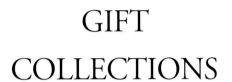

BEACH
BUCKET
WHIMSY

A unique clay pot with wicker handle, stenciled with shells, is outfitted with beach-themed goodies. All the containers are dressed with shells and mirror the cool, refreshing colors of the ocean and the beach landscape. To bring the uplifting quality of the breezes inside, a bottle is filled with scented seashells along with a bath oil and bath salts that will renew the spirit after a long day in the sun. The after-bath splash and sea sponge complete the fun effect for the lucky recipient. Makes a nice house-warming gift.

The Contents

Scented Shells, see "Little Indulgences."
Scented Shells Refresher Oil, instructions follow.
Ocean Breeze Bath Oil, instructions follow.
Refreshing After-Bath Splash, see "Body Fragrancing."
Relaxation Bath Salts w/Scoop, see "Bathing Rituals".
Accessories:
Sea Sponge
Contents Card

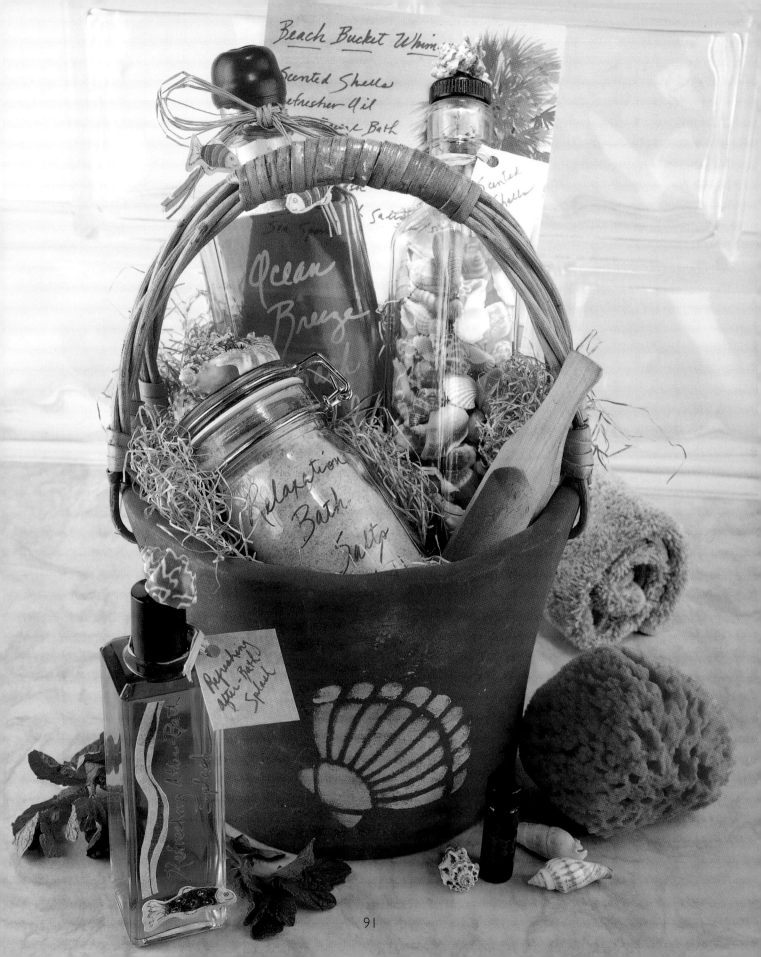

The Presentation

Packaging:

• Place previously scented shells in glass bottle or jar. Cap and glue a shell on the bottle cap. Put a handwritten tag on the bottle with raffia.

• Pour essential oil blend used to scent shells into small, dark glass bottle and label by writing on the side of the bottle with a paint pen.

• Fill decorative bottle with sea shells (enough to line bottom of bottle) then pour Ocean Breeze Bath Oil into bottle. Seal with sealing wax. Tie raffia around the neck of the bottle and hot glue paper fish to the strands of the raffia bow. Write the name of the product on the bottle with a paint pen.

• Fill bottle with Refreshing After-Bath Splash. Glue shell to top of cap. Label with fish sticker and accent piece. Use a paint pen for writing the name of the product on the bottle.

• Fill jar with Relaxation Bath Salts. Glue shells to top of jar. Label by writing on the side of the jar with a paint pen.

Tie scoop to jar with raffia or place the scoop by the salts in the bucket.

• Stencil the clay pot with a template of shells, using an ecru-colored acrylic paint for stenciling. Allow to dry thoroughly before handling. Fill bottom of pot with crumpled paper and top with excelsior or shredded paper. Place products into pot and add sea sponge.

• Write out contents of bucket on separate "beach-themed" paper. Place in pot.

Possible Additions:

• Add a beach towel, flip flops, sunglasses or any item that works well with the theme.

• Add an unscented pillar or votive candle. Suggest that the refresher oil for the shells can also be used to scent the candle. Or buy a ready-made aromatherapy candle in a refreshing or relaxing scent. Just be sure that essential oils were used instead of fragrance (synthetic) oils.

RECIPE

Scented Shells Refresher Oil

This recipe will be enough to make 1/8 oz. If giving as a gift, make two recipes: one for scenting the individual shells; the other for bottling and giving as a refresher oil.

35 drops sweet orange essential oil
15 drops peppermint essential oil
25 drops lavender essential oil

Put all the drops in a 1/8 oz. dark, glass bottle. Label.

RECIPE

Ocean Breeze Bath Oil

Add to the Basic Recipe for Bath Oil (see "Bath Rituals" chapter for recipe):

3 drops of peppermint essential oil
10 drops of sweet orange essential oil
5 drops of sandalwood essential oil
10 drops of lavender essential oil
Base oil: use sweet almond, grapeseed or
a combination of both

In a separate container blend the base oil with the essential oils. Pour into decorative container, cork, and seal.

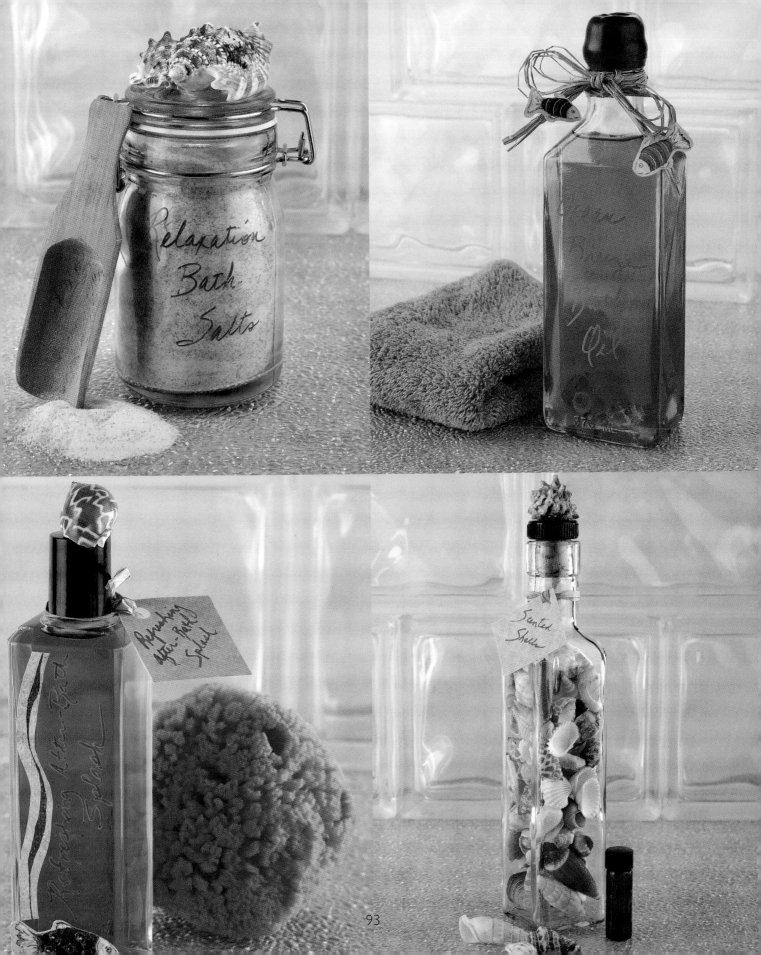

ROMANTIC EVENING BOX

This special box can double as a container for love letters after its contents have been used for one special evening. Blue bottles are used for their exotic look and hold a heavily-scented air spray that will set the tone for romance as well as an aphrodisial massage oil for two. Another glass container holds bath salts - ready for the before-the-massage bath. With some romantic music and perhaps a treat made from the recipes out of the cookbook as well as a lighted aromatherapy candle, it's time to hang the "Do Not Disturb" sign and retreat to a special time together.

The Contents

Romance Is In The Air Room Spray, see "Home Fragrancing."
Romantic Evening Massage Oil, instructions follow.
Exotic Bath Salts, see "Bath Rituals."
Accessories:
Romantic CD or tape
Romantic-theme book, perhaps one on massage for couples
Aromatherapy candle, romantic scent
Do Not Disturb Door Knob, instructions follow

The Presentation

Packaging:
• Pour Romantic Evening Massage Oil into blue glass bottle. Tie with a gold braid ribbon. Label with card stock tag. Use romantic sticker on tag.
• Pour Romance Is in the Air Room Spray into blue glass spray bottle. Tie with a gold braid ribbon. Label with card stock label. Use romantic sticker on tag.
• Put Exotic Bath Salts into attractive glass jar. Tie with gold braid ribbon. Label with card stock tag. Use romantic sticker on tag.
• Make the door sign and add to box.

continued on page 96

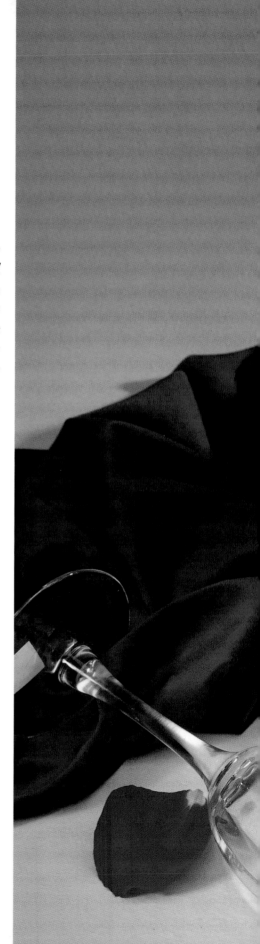

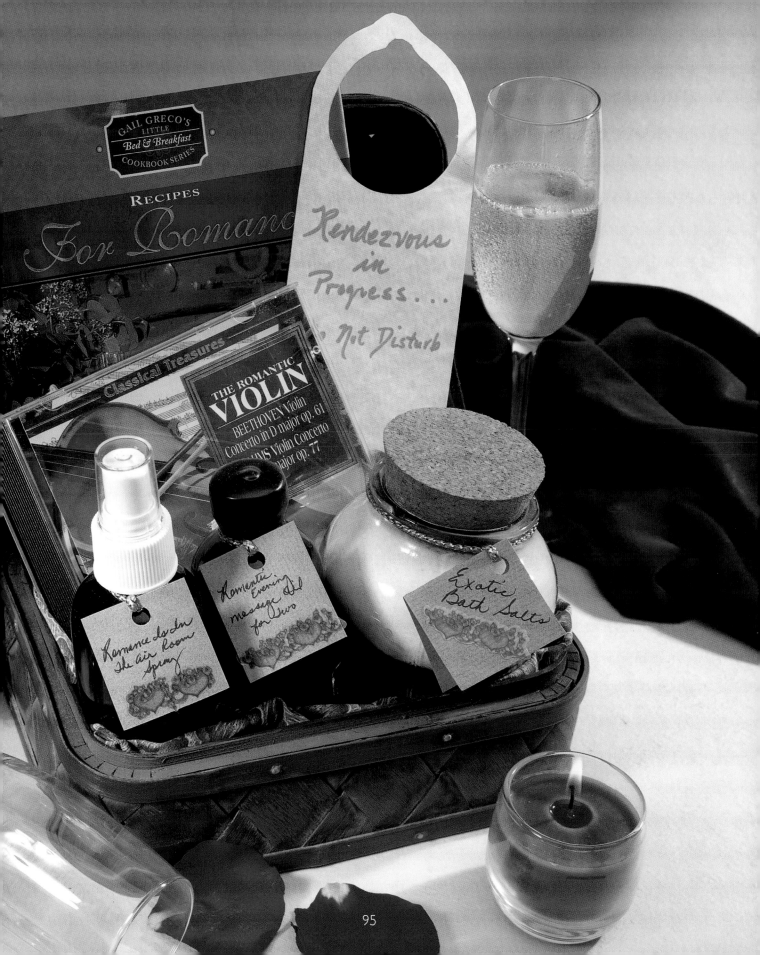

The Presentation (cont.)

The Container:
Find a box that can be used as a gift in itself. The one used in this gift set would make a nice letter or card holder, a jewelry box (perhaps cut a piece of cardboard and wrap it with velvet and use as a filler for the box), or special "couple" memorabilia. The box is lined with a color-coordinated fabric, loosely draped over the bottom of the box.

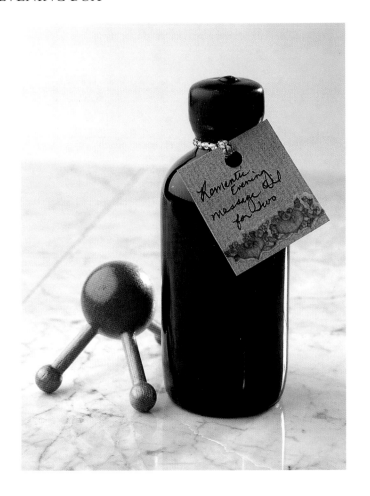

RECIPE

Romantic Evening Massage Oil

2 oz. sweet almond oil (or any appropriate base oil)
10 drops ylang ylang
10 drops jasmine
5 drops sandalwood
5 drops patchouli

Blend well and bottle.

Door Sign

Supplies for one sign:
5" x 11" piece golden tone card stock
Scissors, craft knife, ruler
Romantic theme stencil, stencil brush, burgundy rose acrylic paint.

Instructions:
1. Photocopy the half-pattern given. Fold photocopy on dotted line and cut out for full size. With a craft knife, cut out space for doorknob.
2. Transfer this pattern to card stock. Cut from cardstock.
3. Stencil theme with burgundy rose acrylic paint. Let dry. Add lettering (Rendezvous in Progress - Do Not Disturb) with gold paint pen.

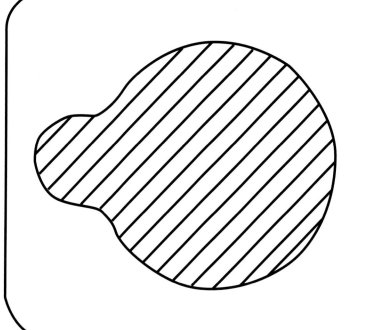

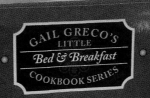
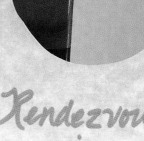
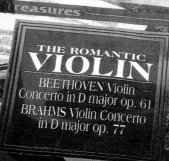

GAIL GRECO'S
LITTLE
Bed & Breakfast
COOKBOOK SERIES

RECIPES

For Roman...

Rendezvous in Progress...

Do Not Disturb

Treasures

THE ROMANTIC
VIOLIN

BEETHOVEN Violin
Concerto in D major op. 61
BRAHMS Violin Concerto
in D major op. 77

HCD-2-3702

ROSE LOVER'S BASKET

A perfect gift for that someone who loves roses and all things scented with rose. This basket is filled with bath items that will soothe and calm even the most frazzled nerves. Add a face cream, a puff and a gift book and voila! A gift basket even someone who doesn't love roses can't resist!

The Contents

Rose Lovers Bath Oil, instructions follow.
Rose Moisturizing Cream, see "Skin Care."
Rose Scented Bath Vinegar, see "Bathing Rituals."
Rose Scented Bath Fizzy, instructions follow.
Accessories:
Bath Puff
Book on Roses
Contents Card

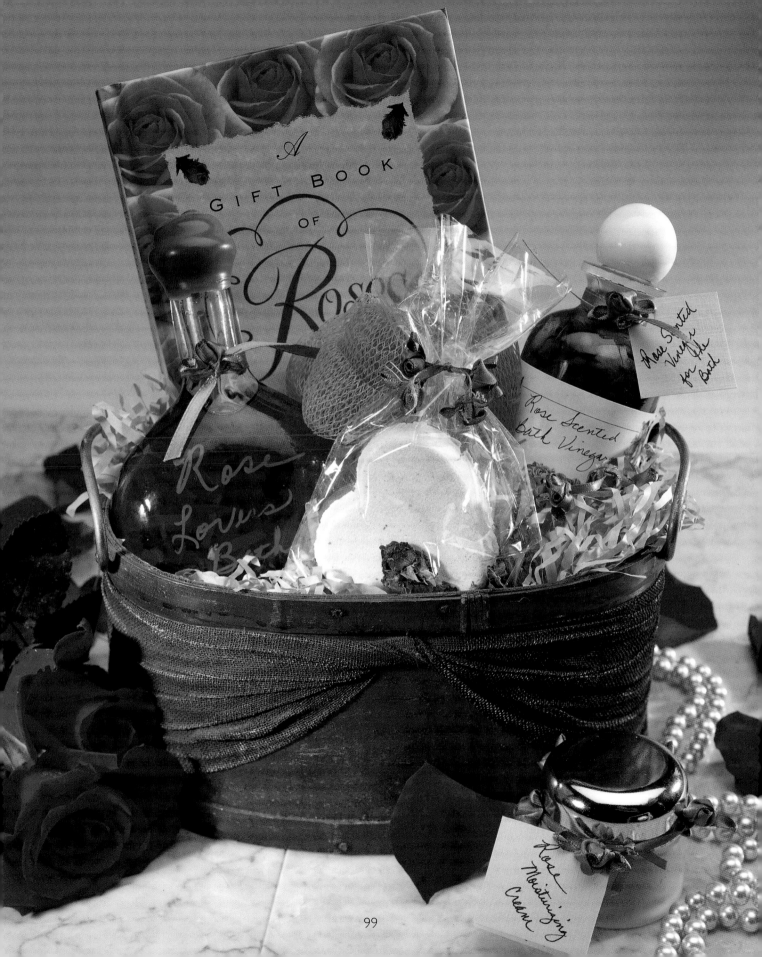

The Presentation

Packaging:

• Put rose buds into decorative glass bottle then pour Rose Lovers Bath Oil into bottle. Cork and seal with sealing wax tinted pink. Tie a pink ribbon around the neck of the bottle. Hot glue a ribbon rose bud on knot of ribbon. Label by writing with pink paint pen directly on the bottle.

• Put Rose Moisturizing Cream into pretty jar. Tie ribbon with roses around top of jar. Label by writing on bottom of jar with pink paint pen and attaching a handwritten tag on pink card stock with the rose ribbon.

• Put rosebuds into bottle (plastic or glass) then pour Rose Scented Bath Vinegar into bottle. Tie a pink ribbon with handwritten tag on pink card stock attached around the neck of the bottle. Hot glue a ribbon rose bud on the knot of the ribbon.

• Place Rose Scented Bath Fizzy and rose buds/petals in cellophane bag. Tie with rose ribbon and place hand-written tag by the bag or it may be attached to the bag.

Additions:

• Add a pretty sheet of stationery on which you've written the contents of the basket and use of the products.

• A Book on Roses is a gift that will remain after the products have been used. Be sure to autograph it with the person's name, your name, the date and occasion, and any special thoughts you may have about the gift recipient.

• Bath Puffs are always a nice addition to a gift basket. Find a complementary color.

The Container:

An oval wooden box, already stained and draped with fabric when purchased, was used. Use pink shredded paper for the filler.

RECIPE

Rose Lovers' Bath Oil

Add to Basic Bath Oil Recipe (see "Bath Rituals" chapter):

10 drops geranium essential oil
15 drops rosewood essential oil
5 drops rose absolute essential oil

Blend well and bottle with dried rose buds.

RECIPE

Rose Scented Bath Fizzy

Add to Basic Bath Fizzy Recipe (see "Bath Ritual" chapter):

15 drops geranium essential oil
5 drops rosewood essential oil
Few drops red food coloring (to make pink color)

Follow the instructions for making Solid Fizzing Bath Salts. Use a heart-shaped soap mold.

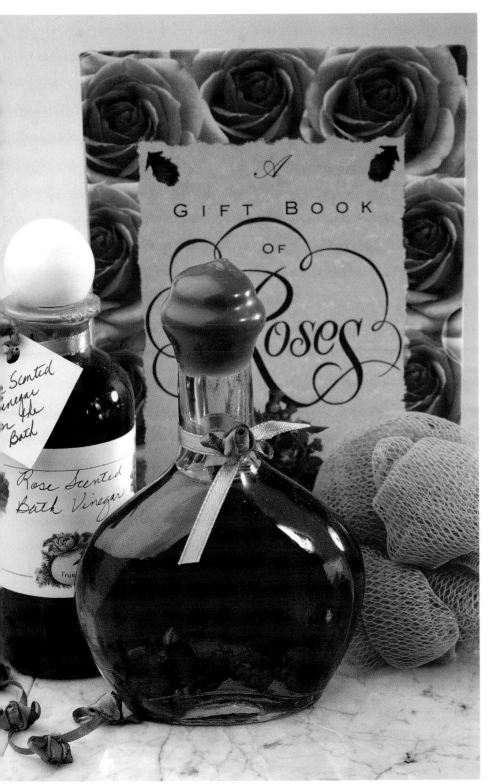

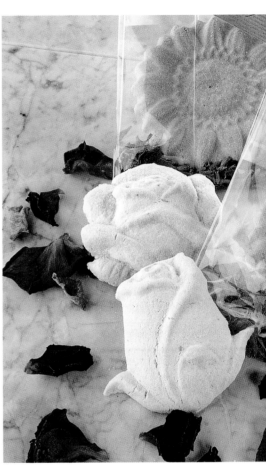

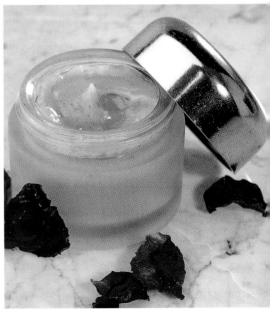

LAVENDER LOVER'S BASKET

Another favorite fragrance is lavender. This basket caters to those who associate wonderful memories to this old-fashioned scent. Stock the basket with wonderful bath items like scented vinegar and bath gel. Add a bath fizzy, a book on herbs, and a special bonus - lavender-scented solid perfume.

The Contents

Lavender Scented Bath Vinegar, see "Bathing Rituals."
Lavender Scented Bath Fizzy, instructions follow.
Lavender Bath and Shower Gel, instructions follow.
Lavender Solid Perfume, see "Body Fragrancing."
Accessories:
Herb Book
Contents Card

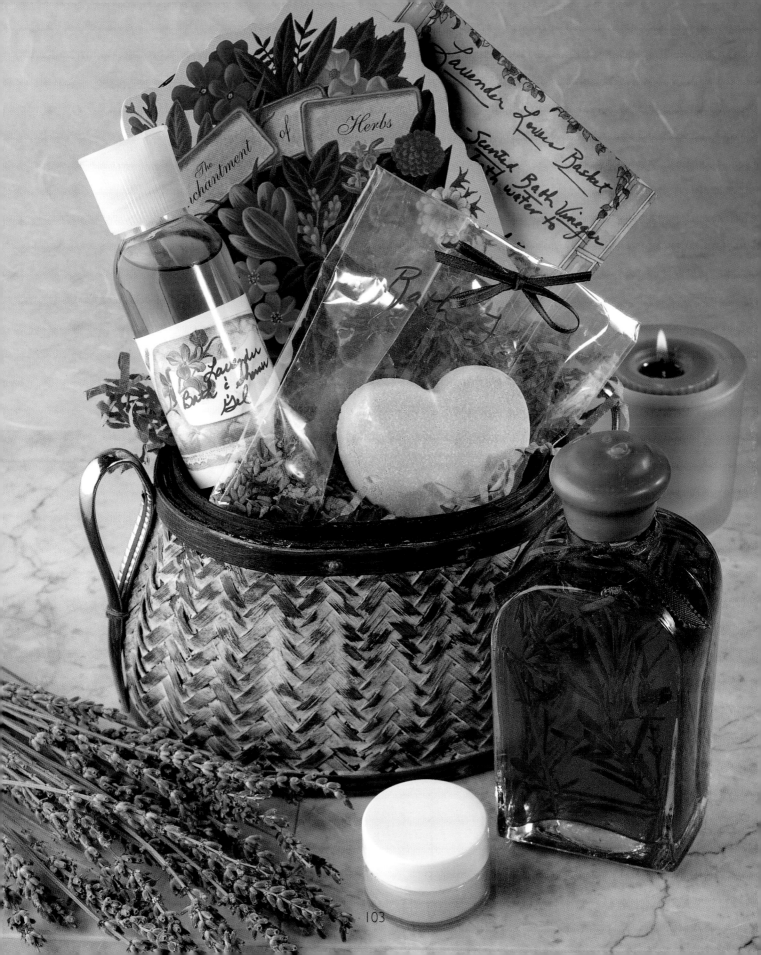

The Presentation

Packaging:

• Put stems of dried lavender in a decorative bottle. Pour Scented Bath Vinegar into the bottle. Cork and seal with sealing wax tinted lavender. Tie a lavender ribbon with card stock tag attached to the neck of the bottle. Write the name of the product directly on the bottle with a lavender paint pen.

• Put the Lavender Bath and Shower Gel in a plastic flip top bottle. Label with ready-made label.

• Place lavender buds and rose petals in plastic bag with Lavender Scented Bath Fizzy. Punch two holes in the top of the bag and put ribbon through them. Tie a bow. Write "Bath Fizzy" on the bag with a paint pen. Insert a usage card in the bag.

• Pour Lavender Solid Perfume into small jars and label by writing on the bottom of the jar. Attach an appropriate flower sticker to the top of the jar.

Additions:

• Write the contents of the basket and usage of the products on a pretty card or a piece of stationery.

• Add a book on lavender or herbs.

The Container:

Find a complementary basket that becomes a gift in itself. This particular basket has a lid and gold arms. It would be a nice container for bath items after the products are used.

RECIPE

Lavender Scented Bath Fizzy

To Basic Bath Fizzy Recipe add:

15 drops lavender essential oil
Few drops red and blue food coloring to make lavender color

Follow the instructions for making Solid Fizzing Bath Salts, (see "Bathing Rituals.") Use a heart-shaped soap mold.

RECIPE

Lavender Bath and Shower Gel

4 oz. unscented bath gel
10 drops lavender essential oil
Few drops of red and blue food coloring to make lavender color

Blend oil and food coloring well with bath gel. Pour into flip top bottle.

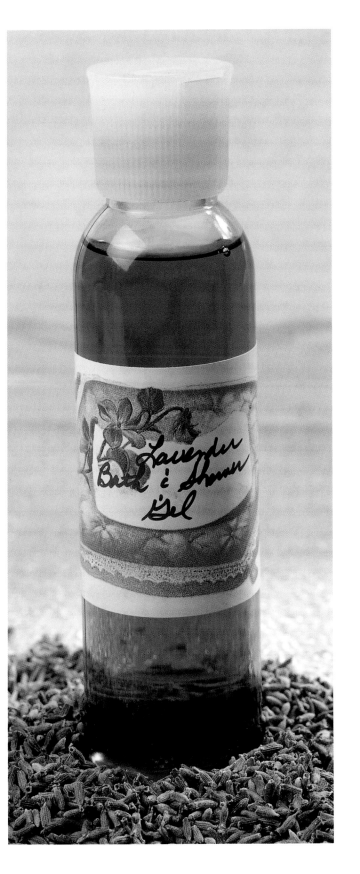

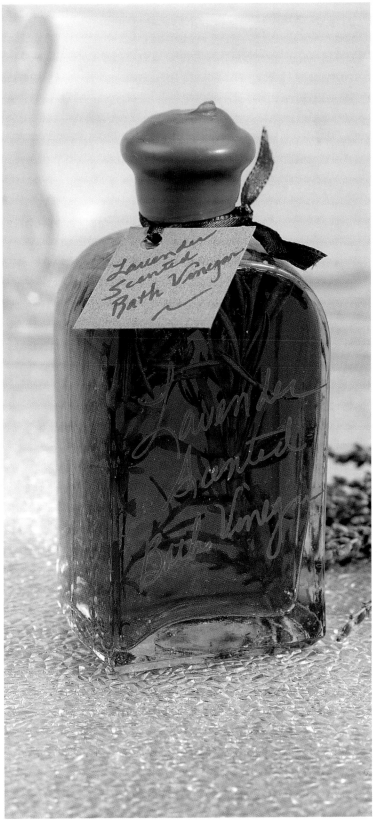

HOLIDAY CHEER BASKET

Ah-h, the cheerful, uplifting smells of Christmas! Capture them in this special basket that accents the pleasure of the holiday with scented pine cones, floating candles, potpourri ornaments, and a room spray to drive the doldrums away after the holidays. Add a special guest towel and the basket is ready to go to someone on your gift list. Makes a great hostess gift.

The Contents

Scented Pine Cones, see "Little Indulgences."
Refresher Oil for Pine Cones, instructions follow.
Winter Blahs Spray, see "Home Fragrancing."
Potpourri Ornaments, instructions follow.
Accessories:
Holiday Towel
Three Floating Star-Shaped Candles
Contents Card

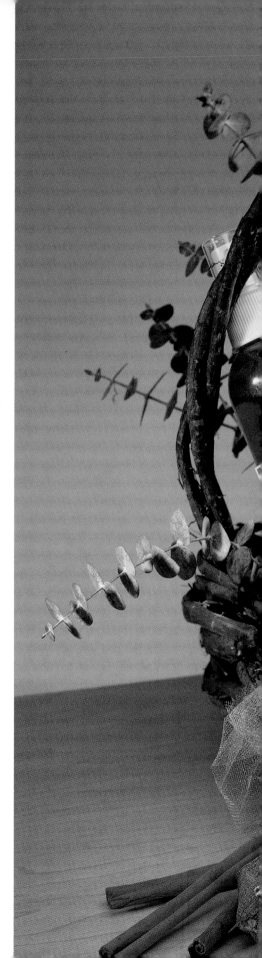

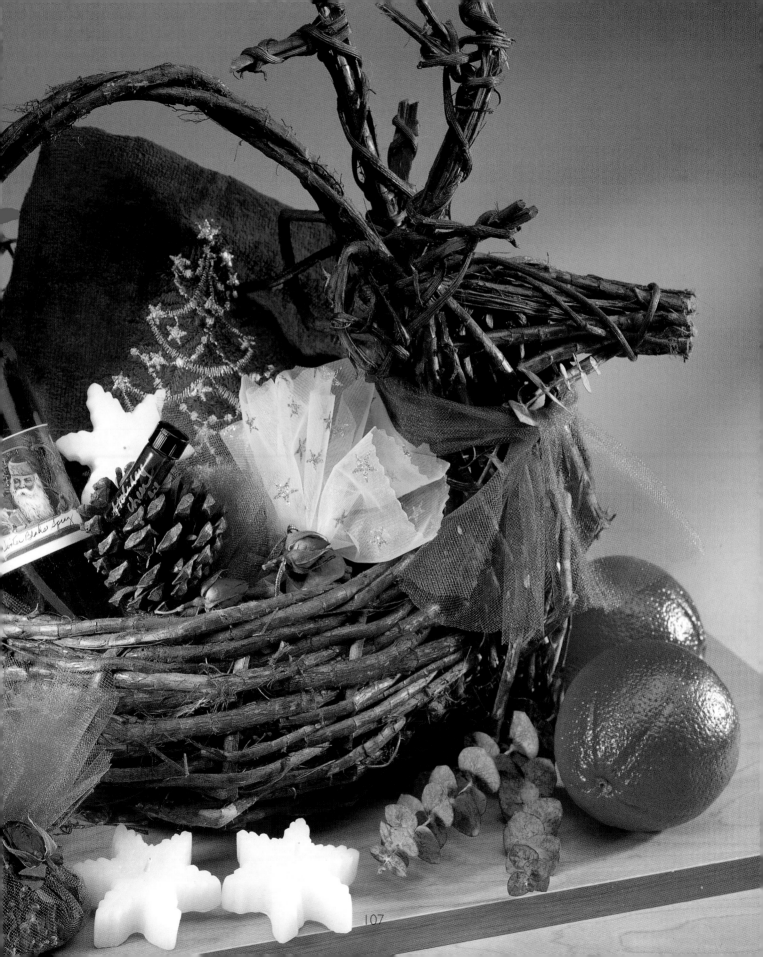

The Presentation

Packaging:

• Place the scented pine cones in the bottom of the basket, leaving a couple out to place among the products.

• Put Holiday Cheer refresher blend in 1/8 oz. bottle with dropper (or add an eye dropper). Write "Holiday Cheer Oil" with paint pen on side of bottle.

• Cut out squares of tulle or netting for Holiday Cheer Potpourri. Place a small amount of potpourri in each square and tie with gold braid ribbon. Decorate each ornament by hot gluing a 1" cinnamon stick, eucalyptus leaf, and rose bud to the front of the ribbon.

• Pour "Winter Blahs" blend into spray bottle – may be plastic or glass. Label with a seasonal ready-made label.

• Write the contents of the basket and the usage of the products on a decorative card.

The Container:

The reindeer basket is a perfect one for this gift set. It will serve as a container for the scented pine cones after the products have been taken out. The scented pine cones serve as the filler along with a piece of gold tulle placed over the top of them under the display. Wrap a gold tulle scarf around the neck of the reindeer.

RECIPE

Holiday Cheer Refresher Oil

30 drops sweet orange
15 drops rosewood
15 drops frankincense
10 drops juniper
5 drops eucalyptus

Place oils in 1/8 oz. dark, glass bottle. Cap tightly and label.
*This recipe may also be used to scent candles.

RECIPE

Holiday Cheer Potpourri

1/2 cup dried juniper berries
1/2 cup dried rose petals
1/2 cup dried eucalyptus leaves
1/2 cup dried orange rind
1/4 cup cinnamon sticks, broken into small pieces
1/8 cup rose hips
1/8 cup cloves
1/8 cup allspice
Dried orange slices
1" cinnamon sticks
Dried rose buds

Combine all but last 3 items of dried materials in large container.

Oils: 3 drops sweet orange essential oil
2 drops rosewood essential oil
2 drops frankincense essential oil
Fixative: 1 tablespoon of orris root or 1/4 oz. oakmoss

Add oils to fixative. Mix with dried materials, adding orange slices, cinnamon sticks and rose buds as a decorative top. Put lid on container and allow to blend for a few days before repackaging.

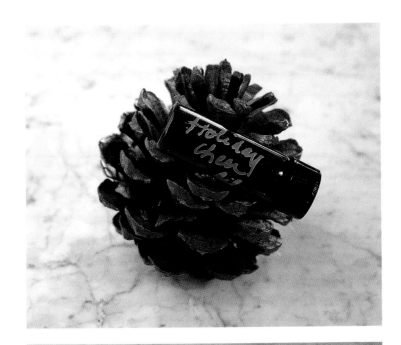

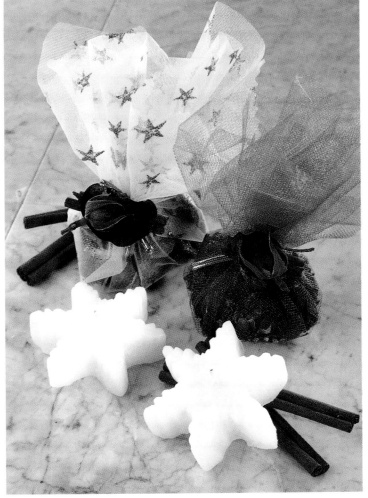

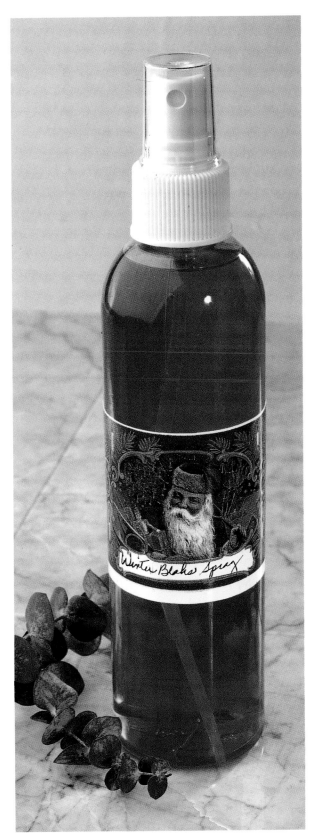

THE ULTIMATE PAMPER ME BASKET

Who deserves a basket filled with a generous sampling of luxurious bath offerings? Maybe it's for a Mother's Day gift, for a birthday or just to cheer someone up. Whatever the occasion, this basket will bring a smile and many hours of pampering for that special person on your list. The list is endless for what might go in to "The Ultimate" pampering gift, but try this assortment to get started.

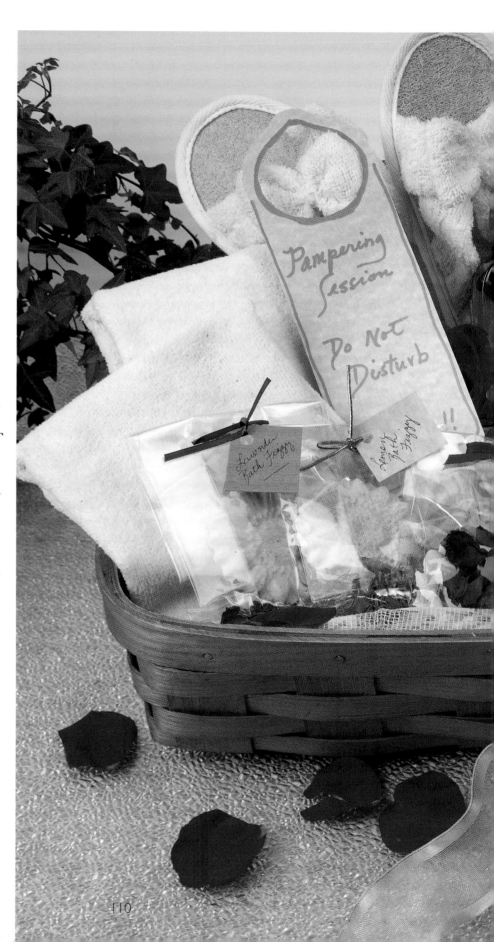

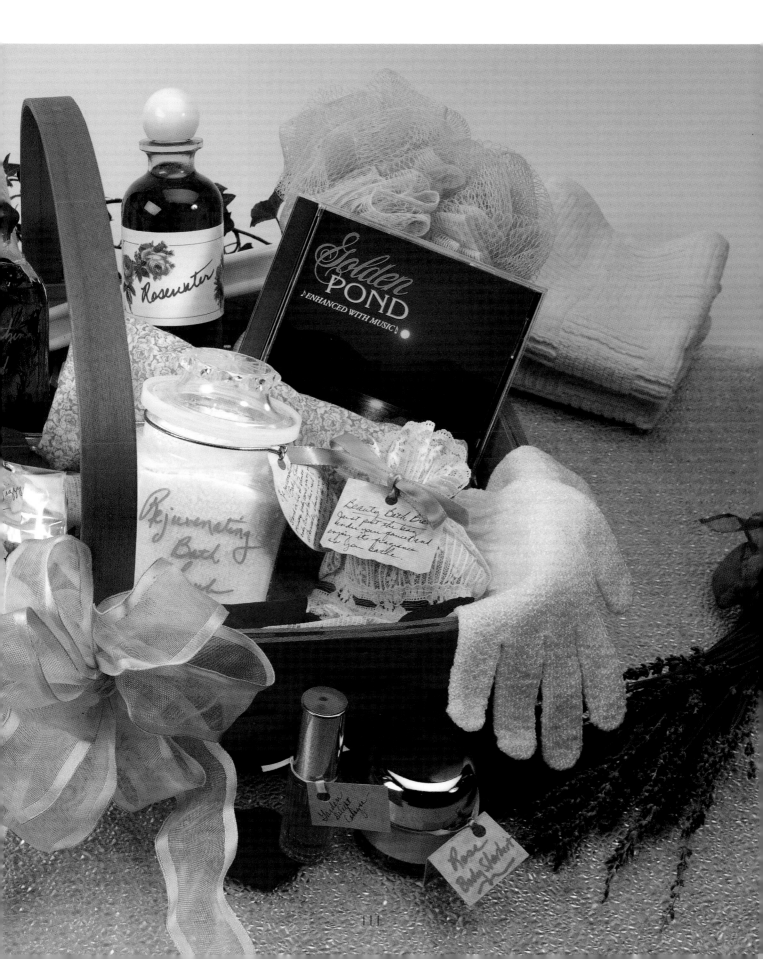

The Contents

Soothing Bath Oil, see "Bathing Rituals."
3 Bath Fizzies (Lemon, Lavender, Rose), see "Bathing Rituals."
Rosewater, see "Skin Care."
Rejuvenating Body Scrub, see "Bathing Rituals."
Rose Body Sherbert, see "Skin Care."
Beauty Bath Brew, instructions follow.
Garden Delight Cologne Spray, see "Body Fragrancing."
Lavender-Scented Compress Bag, see "Healing Routines"

Accessories:
Door sign, see "Romantic Evening Box."
Fancy towel set
Terry cloth slippers
Exfoliating gloves
Bath puff
Meditative CD
Aromatherapy candle or unscented candle with essential oil blend bottle
Terry cloth bath pillow
Contents card

The Presentation

Packaging:
• Put rose buds and lavender pieces in glass bottle. Pour Soothing Bath Oil into the bottle. Cork and seal with sealing wax and pink/gold ribbon. Label by writing on the front of the bottle with a lavender paint pen.
• Place bath fizzies in separate cellophane bags. Put dried lavender buds in with lavender fizzy, dried rose petals in with rose fizzy, and calendula flowers in with the lemon fizzy. Fold over top and use hole puncher to make two holes at top of each bag. Thread color-coordinated ribbons through the holes and tie bow. Attach a handwritten tag to each bag.
• Pour rosewater into a plastic or glass bottle. Label with ready-made label.
• Put Rejuvenating Bath Scrub in apothecary jar - either plastic or glass. Write on front of jar with gold paint pen. Tie a gold braid ribbon around the jar with the tag attached.
• Put the Rose Body Sherbert in a pretty jar and write the name of the product with a paint pen on the bottom of the jar. Place a tag with usage instructions on a ribbon and tie around the top of the jar.
• Package the Beauty Bath Brew in a pretty fabric or lace bag. Attach a usage tag with the bag.
• Put the Garden Delight Cologne in a glass spritzer bottle. Place a tag on a ribbon and tie around the top of the bottle.
• Put the scented flax bag into its outside cover. Insert an instruction sheet on use inside the cover.

• Make the door sign and write: Pampering Session – Do Not Disturb - Sh-h-h!!

Additions:
A number of accessories can fill this basket. Let your imagination – and your budget – be your guide!

The Container:
Select a large, flat basket to hold all the products and accessories. Line the basket with an ecru-colored lace. After positioning contents in the basket, scatter some rose petals on the lace bottom. Tie an ecru-colored bow on the handle of the basket. Attach a hand-made card that lists the contents of the basket and their uses.

RECIPE

Beauty Bath Brew

Combine the following in a container:

1 cup dried chamomile flowers
1/2 cup dried rose petals
1 cup lavender seeds
1/2 cup dried peppermint
1 cup dried lemon verbena

Place in sealable tea bags or small muslin bags.

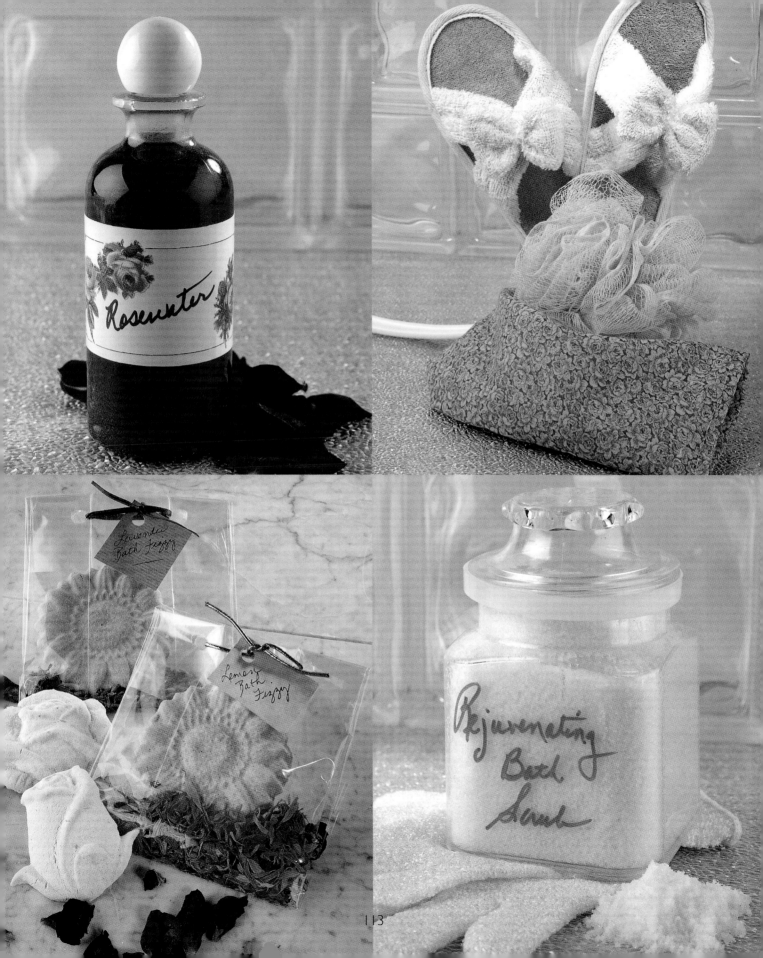

HANDS AND FEET PAMPER BASKET

Here's a basket for everyone! Who wouldn't like pampering products for the two most neglected parts of the body that do more than their share of the work! Load up the basket with all the recipes in this book that pertain to hands and feet, providing instructions on how to rejuvenate tired feet and smooth worn hands. Add a foot massager, socks, gloves, and other accessories to pamper the feet and hands.

The Contents

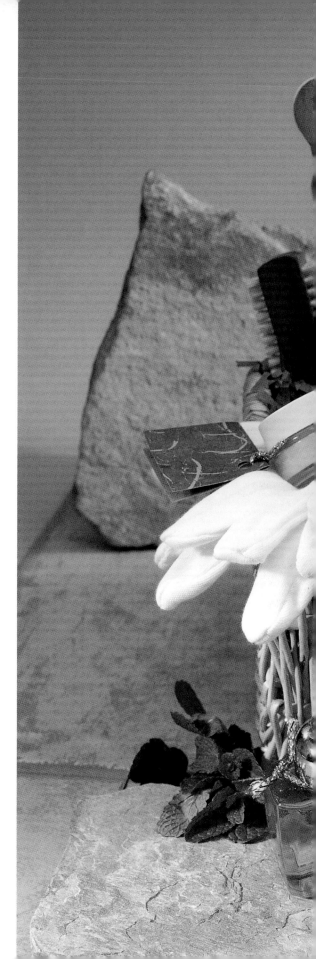

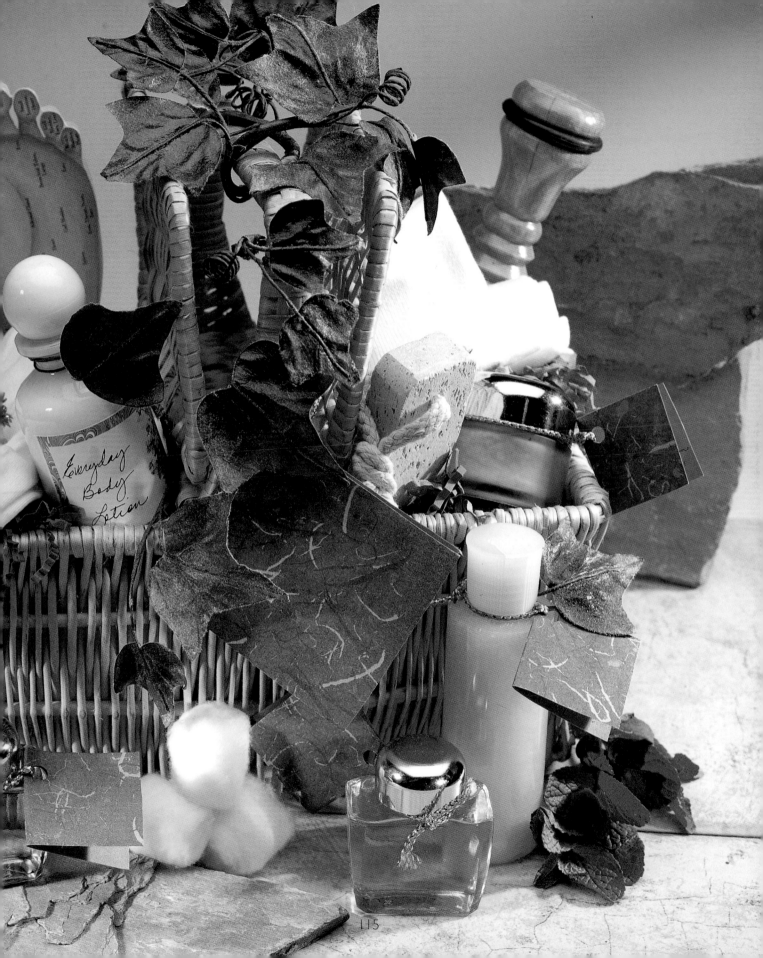

The Presentation

Packaging For Foot Products:

• Pour the Invigorating Foot Bath into flip top plastic container. Label by writing on the bottle with a green paint pen. Attach an instruction tag with gold braid ribbon.

• Pour Perk-Me-Up Oil into small glass jar. Label by writing on the bottle with a green paint pen. Attach an instruction tag with gold braid ribbon.

• Put Overnight Foot Treatment Pomade in a small glass jar. Label by writing on the cap of the jar with a green paint pen. Attach an instruction sheet with gold braid ribbon.

Packaging For Hand Products:

• Put Hand Nourishment Cream in glass jar. Write name of product on bottom of jar. Attach an instruction tag with gold braid ribbon.

• Pour Everyday Body Cream into plastic bottle. Label with ready-made label. Tie one of the faux ivy leaves around top of bottle.

• Pour Nail Soak into small glass bottle. Label by writing on side of bottle with green paint pen. Attach an instruction tag with gold braid ribbon.

The Container:

This particular basket is perfect to do two pamperings since it has hamper openings on each side. Fill the bottom of the basket with crumpled paper, then cover with decorative green or brown (or a combination) shredded paper. Add some faux ivy greenery along the handle and in the basket among the contents. Add a handwritten card tied to the handle with gold braid ribbon.

RECIPE

Strengthening Nail Soak

2 tablespoons castor oil
5 drops essential oil of sandalwood
2 drops tea tree

Combine and pour into small bottle or jar. Refrigerate. Soak fingertips 3 times a week for 5-10 minutes to strengthen dry, brittle, weak nails. Follow with moisturizer.

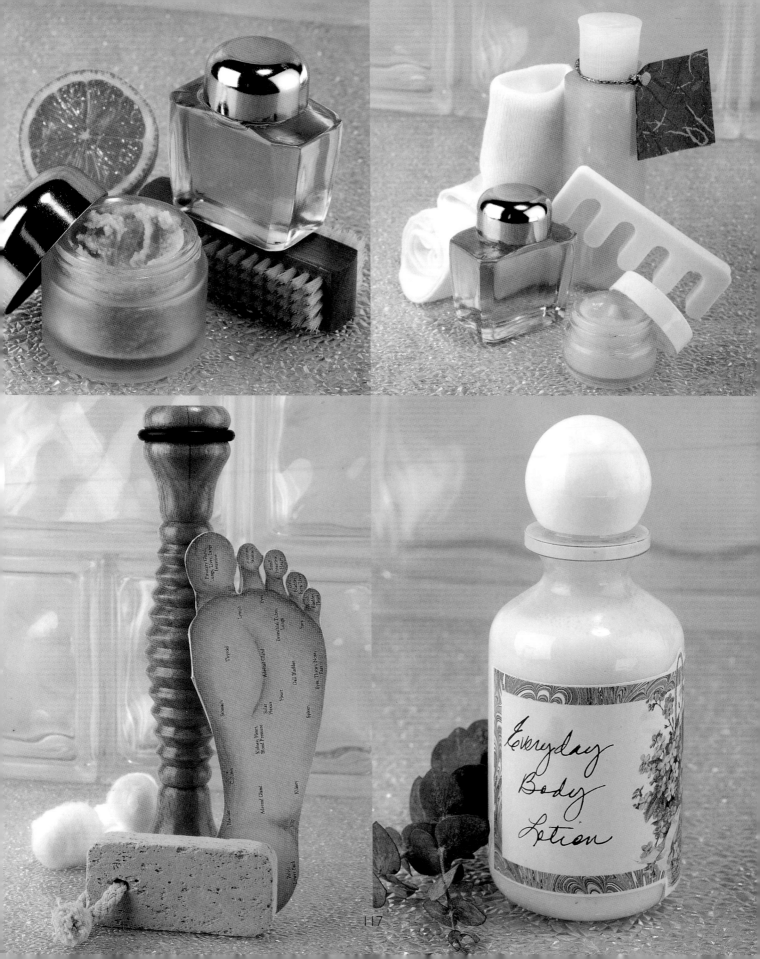

TRAVEL KIT
FOR
PLANE

This is a must-have for friends and family who fly a great deal. Not only does the gift collection include a travel kit that can be taken individually on the trip, but also a number of necessary accessories to make any trip more pleasurable.

The Contents

First Aid Kit w/Cover, instructions follow.
Achy Joints Bath Salts in Envelope, see "Packaging".
Accessories:
Ear Plugs
Inflatable Neck Pillow
Eye Shades
Scented Eye Mask, instructions follow.
Passport Cover
Book on Jet Lag

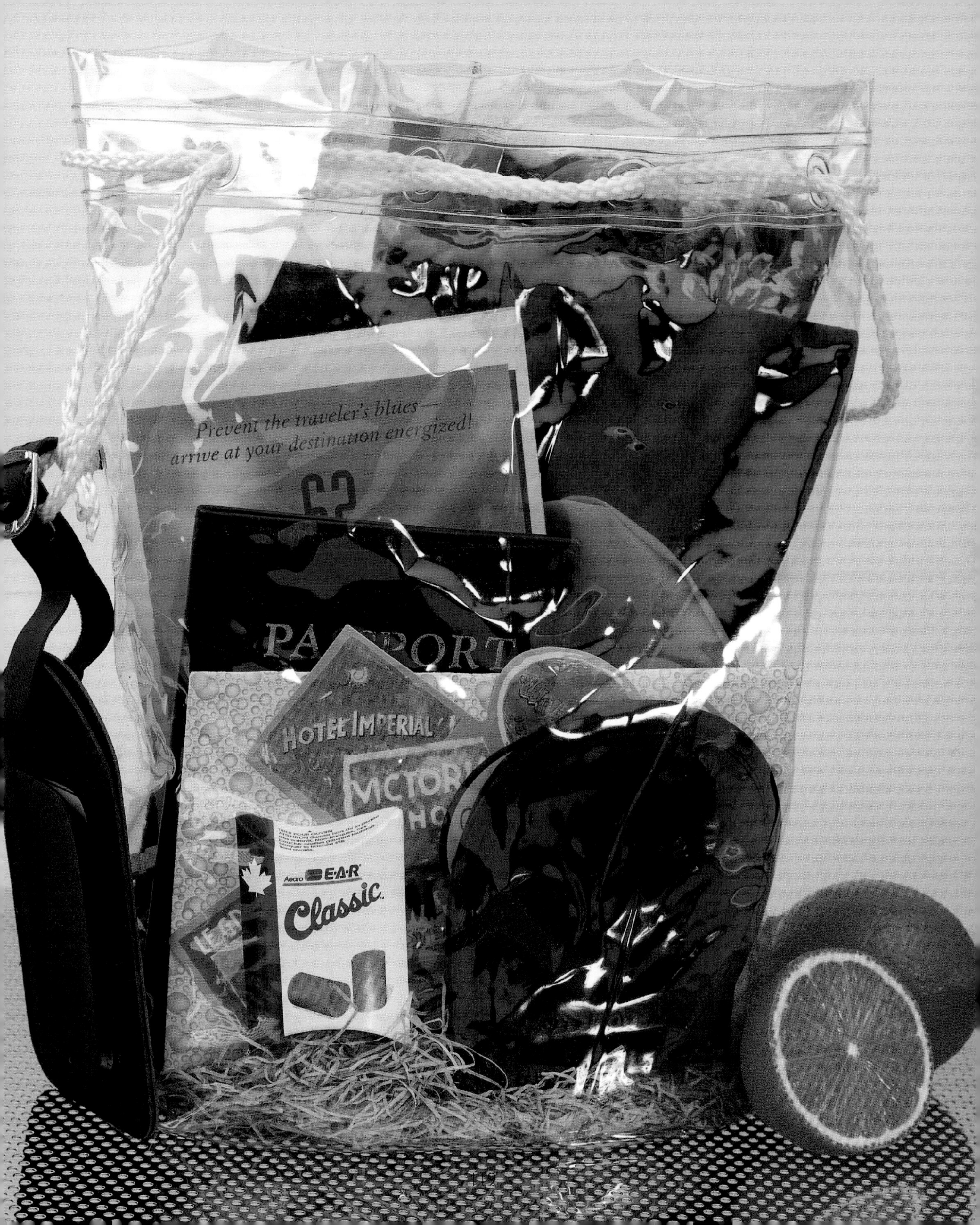
Prevent the traveler's blues—
arrive at your destination energized!
PASSPORT
HOTEL IMPERIAL
Aearo E-A-R
Classic

The Presentation

Packaging:

• A plastic envelope case is used for the First Aid Kit. These can be found in cosmetic areas of retail stores. Follow these instructions for packaging.

Fill each 1/8 oz. dark, glass bottle with one of the following:

> Calming oil, see "Aromatherapy-on-the-Go."
> Uplifting oil, see "Aromatherapy-on-the-Go."
> Tea tree essential oil
> Lavender essential oil
> Eucalyptus essential oil

Label each bottle with its contents by writing on the side with a paint pen (vary colors). Attach a small Velcro® disk to the back of each bottle and its mate to a corresponding space in the plastic envelope case. Press the bottle against the fastener in the case.

Put a carrier/base oil (or combination of several) in a small plastic bottle. Label by writing on the side with a paint pen. Attach a small Velcro® disk to the back of the bottle and follow preceding instructions for attaching to case.

Place the empty plastic spray bottle at the top of the case. It will stay in position when the case is closed. Put Lavender First Aid Ointment (see "Healing Routines.") in small jar. Label by writing on bottom of jar. Attach larger Velcro® disks as described and attach to case.

In the back pocket of the case, insert a cotton hankie. Include a small plastic baggie.
Place an "Aromatherapy First Aid Kit" instruction booklet in the back of the case behind the hankie (see "Aromatherapy on the Go").

• Put Achy Joints Bath Salts in sealable baggie and place in envelope (see "Packaging"). Use a die cut (travel theme) as the label.

The Container:
A heavy-duty plastic bag is just the right container for presenting your gifts and for the recipient to take on the plane. Add a small amount of filler in the bottom of the bag then stock it full of goodies that will ensure a good trip. Add a luggage ID tag to the side to complete the gift.

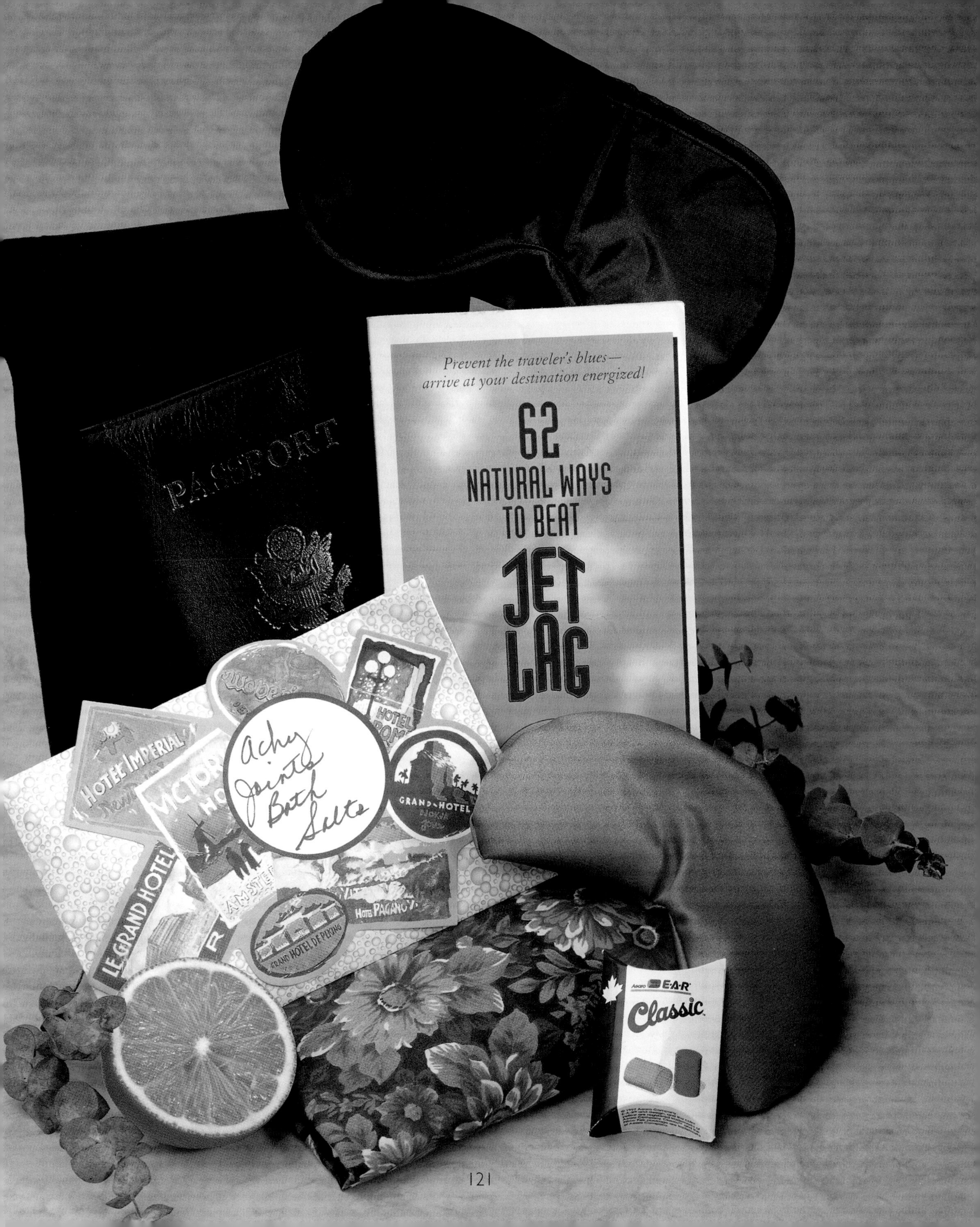

PASSPORT
Prevent the traveler's blues—
arrive at your destination energized!
62
NATURAL WAYS
TO BEAT
JET
LAG
Achy
Joints
Bath
Salts
HOTEL IMPERIAL
LE GRAND HOTEL
GRAND-HOTEL
E·A·R
Classic

TRAVEL KIT FOR CAR

Car travel can be even more pleasant with this travel kit that can go anywhere. The theme of the gift is basically the same as the one for plane travel. One of the differences in this kit is that the spray bottle is filled and ready to be used. Also the type of accessories change in this kit.

The Contents

First Aid Kit w/Cover, see "Travel Kit for Plane."
Soothing Bath Salts in Envelope, instructions follow.
Accessories:
Car Scenter
Book on Tape
CD or music audio tape

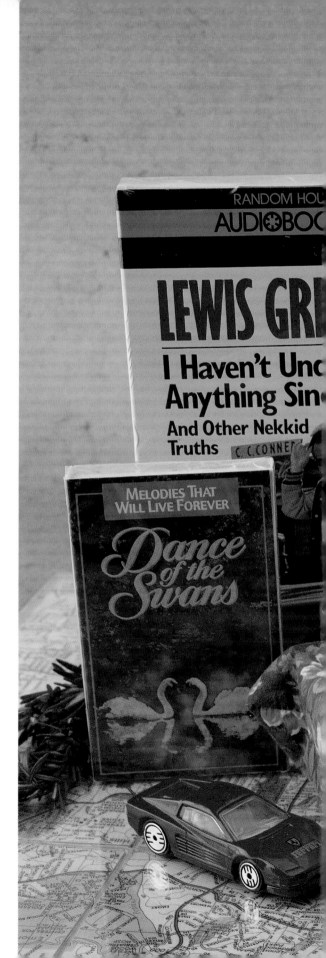

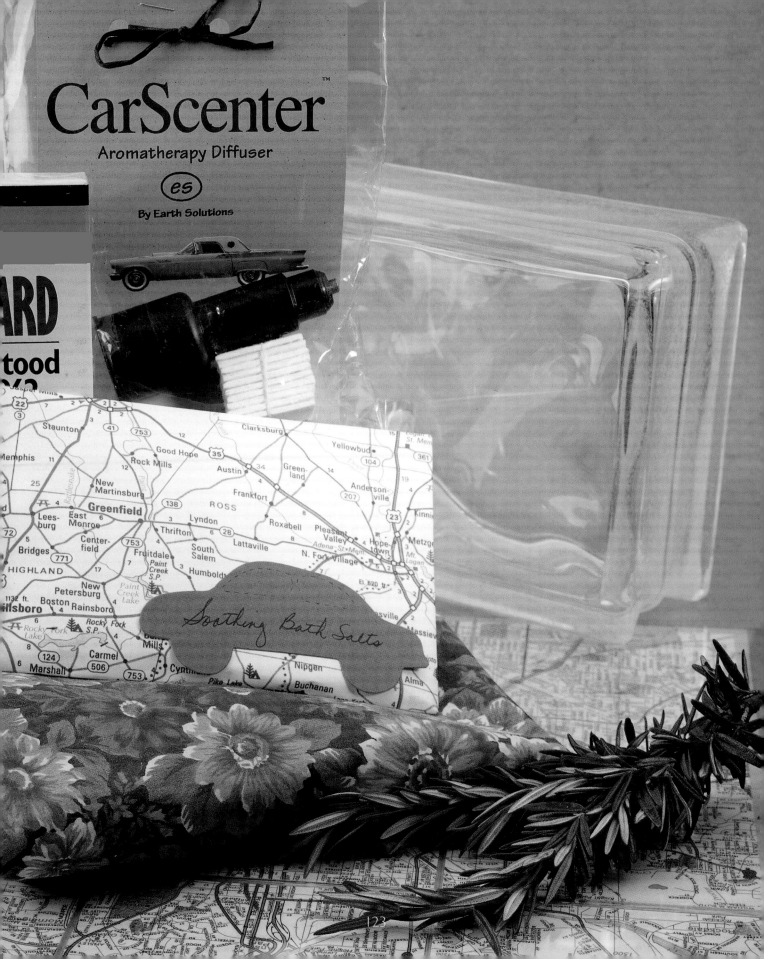

The Presentation

Packaging:

• Follow the instructions in "Travel Kit for Plane" for assembling the first aid kit. Instead of an empty spray bottle, fill the bottle with Long Distance Driving Spray (see "Home Fragrancing").

• Follow instructions for making the envelope in "Travel Kit for Plane." Use any travel scene as the paper for the envelope. Use a die cut of an auto for the label. Put Soothing Bath Salts (instructions follow) in sealable baggie and place in envelope.

The Container:

Use a heavy-duty plastic bag with cord. Arrange items in bag and use a luggage die cut as the label for the container.

RECIPE

Soothing Bath Salts

To Basic Bath Salts Recipe, (see "Bathing Rituals" for recipe) add:

10 drops lavender essential oil
5 drops clary sage essential oil

Blend together and use about 1/4 cup for envelope (enough for one bath).

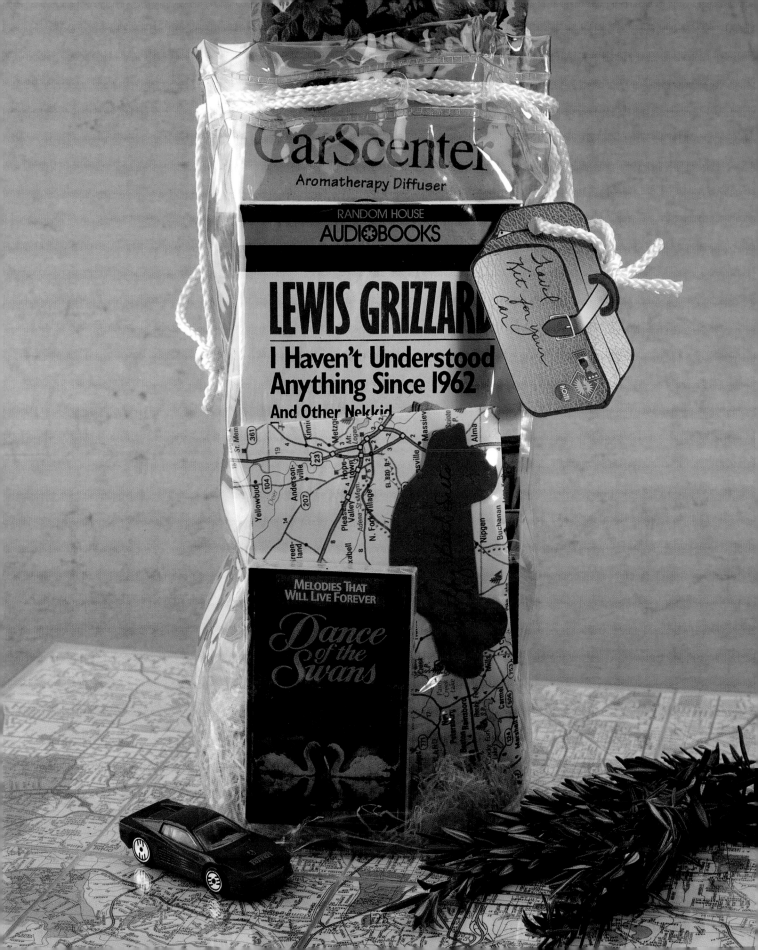

Equivalency Chart

I found an equivalency chart to be a big help when figuring amounts to use in recipes. Keep it close by as a helpful guide.

Drops	Teaspoons	Ounces
25	1/4	
50	1/2	
75	3/4	1/8
150	1 1/2	1/4
	3 (1 T)	1/2
	6 (2 T)	1
	9 (3 T)	1 1/2
	12 (4 T)	2

These measurements aren't always exact, however. Drops from different droppers are not all the same amounts – hole sizes vary and size of dropper varies from smaller to larger bottles. You will need to experiment with the dropper you are using to get a more exact measurement.

Metric Conversion Chart

Sometimes recipes will use metric measurements (especially since there are many intriguing European aromatherapists who have written books). I was stumped as to how to do the recipe until I finally sat down and figured the conversion. It goes like this:

METRIC

1 ml	20 drops
5 ml	1 teaspoon or approximately 100 drops
10 ml	2 teaspoons
15 ml	3 teaspoons (1 tablespoon) or 1/2 oz.
25-30 ml	6 teaspoons (2 tablespoons) or 1 oz.
50-60 ml	2 1/2 tablespoons or 2 oz.
90-100 ml	5 tablespoons or 3 oz.

INCHES TO MILLIMETERS AND CENTIMETERS

Inches	MM	CM
1/8	3	.3
1/4	6	.6
3/8	10	1.0
1/2	13	1.3
5/8	16	1.6
3/4	19	1.9
7/8	22	2.2
1	25	2.5
1-1/4	32	3.2
1-1/2	38	3.8
1-3/4	44	4.4
2	51	5.1
3	76	7.6
4	102	10.2
5	127	12.7
6	152	15.2
7	178	17.8
8	203	20.3
9	229	22.9
10	254	25.4
11	279	27.9
12	305	30.5

INDEX

INDEX